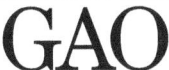

I0470180

September 2012

# PREVENTION AND PUBLIC HEALTH FUND

# Activities Funded in Fiscal Years 2010 and 2011

**To access this report electronically, scan this QR Code.**

Don't have a QR code reader? Several are available for free online.

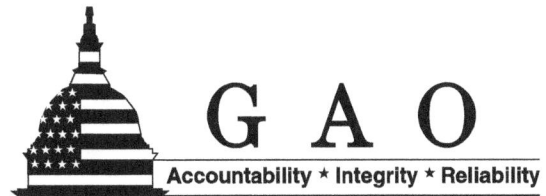

GAO-12-788

# G A O
Accountability * Integrity * Reliability

# Highlights

Highlights of GAO-12-788, a report to congressional requesters

# PREVENTION AND PUBLIC HEALTH FUND

## Activities Funded in Fiscal Years 2010 and 2011

## Why GAO Did This Study

In March 2010, PPACA established the PPHF to provide for expanded and sustained national investment in prevention and public health programs, including prevention research, health screenings, and immunization programs. PPACA appropriated $500 million for fiscal year 2010, $750 million for fiscal year 2011, and additional amounts for future fiscal years to operationalize the PPHF.

HHS allocates funding from the PPHF for specific prevention and public health activities administered by HHS agencies. The agencies, once funds are transferred to them, use the PPHF funds to support individual projects through, for example, grants and contracts. GAO was asked to provide information on how PPHF funds were allocated for fiscal years 2010 and 2011. This report describes, for those fiscal years, (1) the HHS agencies and activities for which PPHF allocations were made, (2) the process and criteria HHS used to allocate PPHF funds, and (3) HHS reporting of the outcomes of activities receiving PPHF funding. GAO reviewed agency documents, including budget justifications, funding announcements, data on PPHF allocations and awards of PPHF-funded grants, contracts, and interagency agreements; examined agency websites; and interviewed HHS officials.

HHS provided technical comments on a draft of this report, which were incorporated as appropriate.

View GAO-12-788. For more information, contact Katherine Iritani at (202) 512-7114 or iritanik@gao.gov.

## What GAO Found

For fiscal years 2010 and 2011, the Department of Health and Human Services (HHS) allocated funds from the Prevention and Public Health Fund (PPHF) for 43 activities in five agencies. These activities—which include HHS programs and initiatives—were administered by HHS's Agency for Healthcare Research and Quality (AHRQ), Centers for Disease Control and Prevention (CDC), Health Resources and Services Administration (HRSA), Substance Abuse and Mental Health Services Administration (SAMHSA), and the Office of the Secretary (OS). Most of the $500 million available for fiscal year 2010 was allocated for activities administered by HRSA, and most of the $750 million available for fiscal year 2011 was allocated for activities administered by CDC (see fig.). HHS agencies funded individual projects with PPHF funds through grants, contracts, and interagency agreements.

**Prevention and Public Health Fund (PPHF) Allocations by HHS Agency, Fiscal Years 2010 and 2011**

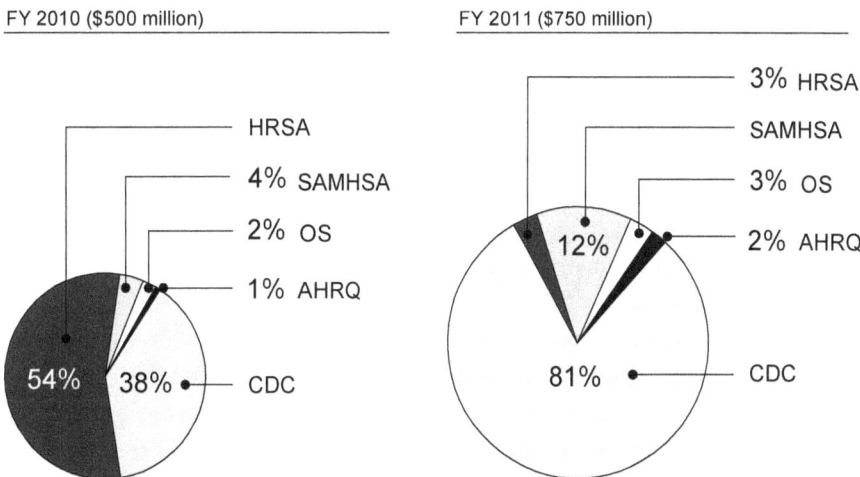

FY 2010 ($500 million)

- HRSA
- 4% SAMHSA
- 2% OS
- 1% AHRQ
- 54%
- 38% CDC

FY 2011 ($750 million)

- 3% HRSA
- SAMHSA
- 3% OS
- 2% AHRQ
- 12%
- 81% CDC

Source: GAO analysis of HHS information.

Note: Percentages do not total to 100% due to rounding.

Because the PPHF was established midway through fiscal year 2010 and after the President had submitted the fiscal year 2011 budget request, for the fund's first 2 years HHS used an abbreviated process to allocate PPHF funds. Instead of developing HHS-wide written criteria, HHS requested that its agencies propose activities for PPHF funding based on language in the Patient Protection and Affordable Care Act (PPACA) provision establishing the PPHF. According to HHS, the proposed activities were also aligned with existing departmental priorities.

HHS has relied on its agencies to establish performance measures and targets and to track outcomes (the results) of the PPHF-funded activities. Agency officials reported that for many activities, it is too early to report outcomes because many projects receiving PPHF funding in fiscal years 2010 and 2011 are multiyear projects or have not yet completed evaluations.

_____ **United States Government Accountability Office**

# Contents

Tables

Figures

## Abbreviations

| | |
|---|---|
| AHRQ | Agency for Healthcare Research and Quality |
| ASFR | Office of the Assistant Secretary for Financial Resources |
| CDC | Centers for Disease Control and Prevention |
| FOA | funding opportunity announcement |
| GPRA | Government Performance and Results Act |
| HHS | Department of Health and Human Services |
| HRSA | Health Resources and Services Administration |
| OS | Office of the Secretary |
| PPACA | Patient Protection and Affordable Care Act |
| PPHF | Prevention and Public Health Fund |
| SAMHSA | Substance Abuse and Mental Health Services Administration |

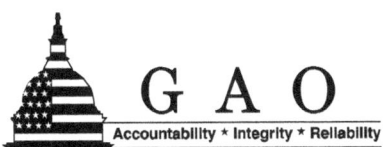

**United States Government Accountability Office**
**Washington, DC 20548**

September 13, 2012

The Honorable Orrin G. Hatch
Ranking Member
Committee on Finance
United States Senate

The Honorable Tom Coburn
Ranking Member
Permanent Subcommittee on Investigations
Committee on Homeland Security and Governmental Affairs
United States Senate

In March 2010, the Patient Protection and Affordable Care Act (PPACA) established the Prevention and Public Health Fund (PPHF) to provide for expanded and sustained national investment in prevention and public health programs, such as prevention research, health screenings, and immunization programs.[1] PPACA appropriated $500 million to the fund for fiscal year 2010, $750 million for fiscal year 2011, a total of $3.75 billion for fiscal years 2012 through 2014, and $2 billion for fiscal year 2015 and each subsequent fiscal year.[2]

For each fiscal year since the passage of PPACA, the Department of Health and Human Services (HHS) has allocated PPHF funds—that is, established a plan for funding specific prevention and public health-related activities—for that year and then transferred funds from the PPHF to the appropriation accounts for the HHS agencies that administer these

---

[1]Pub. L. No. 111-148, §§ 4002, 10401(b). 124 Stat. 119, 541, 974 (2010).

[2]More recently, the Middle Class Tax Relief and Job Creation Act of 2012 amended this provision, reducing the annual amounts appropriated for the PPHF in fiscal years 2013-2021. Pub. L. No. 112-96, § 3205, 126 Stat. 156, 194.

activities.[3] Once HHS has allocated and transferred PPHF funds, HHS agencies use PPHF funding for individual projects to carry out the activities through, for example, grant and contract awards.[4]

You asked us to provide detailed information on the allocation of PPHF funding for fiscal years 2010 and 2011, including how decisions were made to allocate PPHF funding for specific HHS activities, the entities receiving PPHF funding, and the outcomes—that is, the results—of those activities. This report describes (1) the HHS agencies and activities for which PPHF funding was allocated for fiscal years 2010 and 2011 and the entities receiving PPHF funding, (2) the process and criteria HHS used to allocate and award PPHF funds for fiscal years 2010 and 2011, and (3) HHS reporting of the performance measures, targets, and outcomes of activities and projects receiving PPHF funding.

To describe the HHS agencies and activities for which PPHF funding was allocated and for which awards were made for fiscal years 2010 and 2011, we reviewed documents, such as budget justifications, funding opportunity announcements, and data on PPHF allocations and recipients of PPHF-funded grants, contracts, and interagency agreements provided by HHS agencies. We also interviewed officials from the Office of the Assistant Secretary for Financial Resources (ASFR) within the HHS Office of the Secretary (OS), which is involved in the allocation of PPHF funds, and HHS agencies and the OS (hereafter collectively referred to as

---

[3]Such activities include the Community Transformation Grants program and the National Prevention Strategy. The Community Transformation Grants program, established under PPACA and administered by HHS's Centers for Disease Control and Prevention (CDC), awards competitive grants to state and local governmental agencies and community-based organizations for activities that reduce chronic disease rates, prevent the development of secondary conditions, address health disparities, and develop a stronger evidence base of effective prevention programming. Pub. L. No. 111-148, §§ 4201, 10403, 124 Stat. 564, 975 (2010). Because CDC refers to this program as the "Community Transformation Grants program", we use that name in referring to the program in this report. The National Prevention Strategy was developed by the National Prevention Council, which is composed of the heads of 17 federal agencies that consulted with outside experts and stakeholders. The strategy, released in June 2011, includes actions that public and private partners can take to help Americans stay healthy and fit.

[4]Throughout this report we use the following terms: "agency" to refer to agencies within HHS and the Office of the Secretary; "activity" to refer to HHS programs and initiatives, such as the National Prevention Strategy; "project" to refer to the specific grants, contracts, or interagency agreements made by a given activity, such as grants for tobacco prevention projects; and "award recipient" to refer to those awarded grants, contracts, and cooperative agreements, such as a state or local government.

HHS agencies) that administered activities that received PPHF funding in fiscal years 2010 and 2011. We summarized funding data HHS reported to us and did not independently verify the reported data. Through our review of the relevant documentation, our discussions with HHS officials, and quality control checks we performed on the data, we determined that the data provided were sufficiently reliable for our purposes. To describe the criteria and processes HHS used to allocate PPHF funds we interviewed HHS and agency officials who were knowledgeable about the decision-making process and reviewed available documentation, including HHS websites. When documentation of the criteria and processes was not available, we report HHS officials' descriptions. To describe how HHS and agencies reported the performance measures, targets, and outcomes of activities and projects receiving PPHF funding, we reviewed HHS's websites, budget justifications, and other documents and interviewed HHS and agency officials. We examined performance measures that HHS established for PPHF-funded activities, the targets set for those activities, and the available information from HHS on outcomes. For all three objectives we also examined relevant laws and other documents related to PPHF allocations and oversight.

We conducted this performance audit from December 2011 to September 2012 in accordance with generally accepted government auditing standards. Those standards require that we plan and perform the audit to obtain sufficient, appropriate evidence to provide a reasonable basis for our findings and conclusions based on our audit objectives. We believe that the evidence obtained provides a reasonable basis for our findings and conclusions based on our audit objectives.

## Background

PPACA established the PPHF to provide for expanded and sustained national investment in prevention and public health programs to improve health and help restrain the rate of growth in private and public sector health care costs.[5] For this purpose, the Secretary of Health and Human Services is required to transfer amounts from the PPHF to HHS accounts to increase funding, over the fiscal year 2008 level, for programs authorized by the Public Health Service Act, "for prevention, wellness, and public health activities including prevention research, health screenings, and initiatives, such as the Community Transformation grant

---

[5]Pub. L. No. 111-148, § 4002(a), 124 Stat. 541.

program, the Education and Outreach Campaign Regarding Preventive Benefits, and immunization programs."[6] Within HHS, agencies including the Agency for Healthcare Research and Quality (AHRQ), the Centers for Disease Control and Prevention (CDC), the Health Resources and Services Administration (HRSA), the Substance Abuse and Mental Health Services Administration (SAMHSA), and the OS administer programs authorized by the Public Health Service Act.

PPACA appropriated $5 billion to the PPHF for fiscal years 2010 through 2014, and $2 billion for each fiscal year thereafter.[7] In February 2012, the Middle Class Tax Relief and Job Creation Act of 2012[8] amended PPACA, reducing the amounts appropriated to the PPHF for fiscal years 2013 through 2021 by a total of $6.25 billion (see table 1).

---

[6]Pub. L. No 111-148, §§ 4002 (c), 10401(b), 124 Stat. 541, 974. Because CDC refers to the "Community Transformation Grants program", we use that name in referring to the program in this report. PPACA provided for the implementation of the Education and Outreach Campaign Regarding Preventive Benefits—a national public-private partnership for a prevention and health promotion outreach and education campaign to raise public awareness of health improvement across the lifespan. Pub. L. No. 111-148, § 4004, 124 Stat. 544 (2010).

[7]Pub. L. No. 111-148, § 4002(b), 124 Stat. 541.

[8]Pub. L. No. 112-96, § 3205, 126 Stat. 156, 194.

Table 1: PPACA Appropriations to the PPHF, Fiscal Years 2010-2022

| Fiscal year | PPACA March 2010[a] (in millions) | PPACA as amended February 2012[b] (in millions) | Decrease (in millions) |
|---|---|---|---|
| 2010 | $500 | $500 | — |
| 2011 | 750 | 750 | — |
| 2012 | 1,000 | 1,000 | — |
| 2013 | 1,250 | 1,000 | $250 |
| 2014 | 1,500 | 1,000 | 500 |
| 2015 | 2,000 | 1,000 | 1,000 |
| 2016 | 2,000 | 1,000 | 1,000 |
| 2017 | 2,000 | 1,000 | 1,000 |
| 2018 | 2,000 | 1,250 | 750 |
| 2019 | 2,000 | 1,250 | 750 |
| 2020 | 2,000 | 1,500 | 500 |
| 2021 | 2,000 | 1,500 | 500 |
| 2022 + annually | 2,000 | 2,000 | — |
| **Total fiscal years 2010-2022** | **$21,000** | **$14,750** | **$6,250[c]** |

Source: GAO analysis.

[a]Amounts appropriated by PPACA, Pub. L. No. 111-148, § 4002(b).

[b]Amounts appropriated by PPACA, as amended by Pub. L. No. 112-96, § 3205.

[c]$6.25 billion represents a 37 percent reduction of the amount appropriated to the PPHF for fiscal years 2013 through 2021.

When appropriations are made available, an agency may obligate funds through such actions as awarding discretionary grants, cooperative agreements,[9] or contracts, or through entering into interagency agreements.[10] For discretionary grants,[11] agencies announce the availability of funds through a publicly available notice called a funding

---

[9]A cooperative agreement is an arrangement that has greater agency involvement than a grant. For the purposes of this report, the term grant is used to mean both grants and cooperative agreements. See 31 U.S.C. §§ 6304 (using grant agreements) and 6305 (using cooperative agreements).

[10]In this report we refer to the amount obligated under a grant, cooperative agreement, contract, or interagency agreement as the "amount awarded."

[11]Unlike a formula grant that is based on a precise formula specified in legislation, an agency makes discretionary grant awards on the basis of a competitive process.

GAO-12-788 Prevention and Public Health Fund

opportunity announcement.[12] The funding announcements provide guidance on how to apply for available funding and often identify restrictions on eligibility, such as limiting applicants to states, local governments, tribal organizations, or academic institutions. Funding opportunity announcements also indicate the type of grant award, such as new, continuation, or supplemental. A new grant provides funding for a project that is currently not receiving financial support, a continuation grant provides additional funding for one or more budget periods to a project that would otherwise end, and a supplemental grant increases funding for an approved project during a current budget period.

An agency may also provide federal funding pursuant to a contract, a legal instrument that establishes a binding relationship between the agency and another entity for acquisition of property or services.[13] Agencies can also enter into interagency agreements to carry out projects when, for example, another agency has expertise in an area or has additional capacity to do the work.

---

[12]HHS agencies typically publically announce funding opportunities on www.grants.gov. Each funding announcement is identified by a number assigned by the agency and provides such information as the project purpose, eligibility, evaluation criteria, funding preferences or priorities, and legislative authority. Funding opportunity announcements may also be referred to as request for applications, program announcements, notices of funding availability, or solicitations depending on the agency and type of program—we refer to all types of funding announcements as funding opportunity announcements in this report.

[13]See 31 U.S.C. § 6303. HHS agencies typically publically announce contract solicitations on www.fbo.gov.

The Consolidated Appropriations Act, 2012 required HHS to establish a website that provides information on the use of PPHF funds. Specifically, it required HHS to post on a website specific information relating to use of fiscal year 2012 PPHF funds.[14]

# HHS Agencies and Activities for Which PPHF Funds Were Allocated and Entities That Received PPHF Funding, Fiscal Years 2010 and 2011

HHS allocated PPHF funds for 43 activities in five HHS agencies—AHRQ, CDC, HRSA, OS, and SAMHSA—in the first 2 years of the fund.[15] The majority of the $500 million in PPHF funding available for fiscal year 2010 was allocated for activities administered by HRSA, while the majority of the $750 million in PPHF funding available for fiscal year 2011 was allocated for activities administered by CDC (see fig. 1).

[14]Pub. L. No. 112-74, § 220, 125 Stat. 786, 1085-6 (2011). The provision required HHS to post on the PPHF website specific information on fiscal year 2012 PPHF funds including information on the program or activity receiving funds (to be posted no later than the day after the transfer is made), identification of each grant, cooperative agreement, or contract with a value of $25,000 or more awarded using PPHF funds (to be posted no later than 5 days of the award), as well as annual and semiannual reporting requirements. The President's budget request for fiscal year 2013 requested that the PPHF reporting requirements be rescinded, but as of May 25, 2012, legislation had not been introduced to do so. The Consolidated Appropriations Act, 2012, also contained a provision specifically prohibiting the use of PPHF funds for publicity or propaganda or other expenses related to activities designed to influence the enactment of legislation, regulations, administrative actions, or executive orders before Congress or state or local bodies. See Pub. L. No. 112-74, § 503, 125 Stat. 1110.

[15]According to HHS officials, an activity can consist of a single program, such as CDC's Community Transformation Grants program, or multiple programs, such as SAMHSA's Suicide Prevention activity, which consists of four suicide prevention programs.

**Figure 1: PPHF Allocations by HHS Agency, Fiscal Years 2010 and 2011**

FY 2010 ($500 million)    FY 2011 ($750 million)

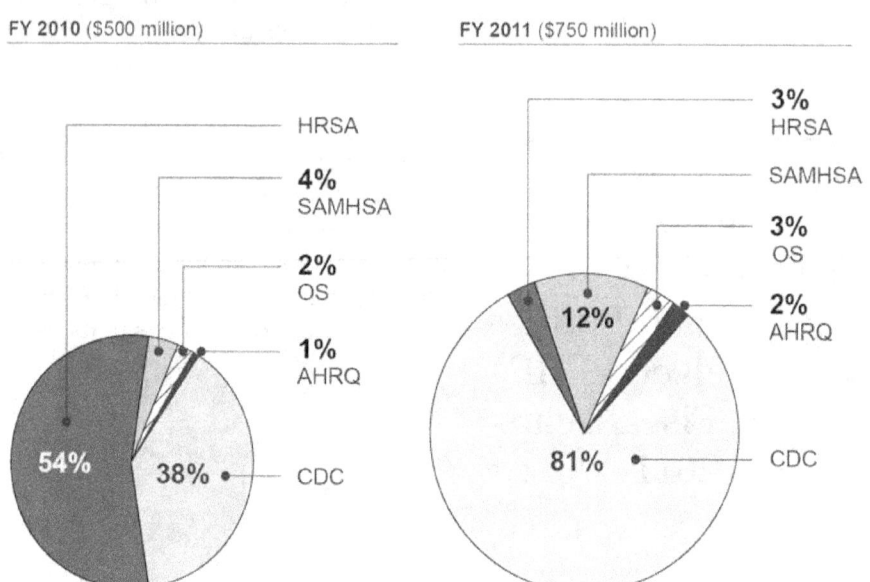

Source: GAO analysis of HHS information.

Note: This figure summarizes HHS information on fiscal year (FY) 2010 and 2011 PPHF allocations to activities administered by five HHS agencies—the Agency for Healthcare Research and Quality (AHRQ), the Centers for Disease Control and Prevention (CDC), the Health Resources and Services Administration (HRSA), the Substance Abuse and Mental Health Services Administration (SAMHSA), and the Office of the Secretary (OS). Percentages do not total to 100% due to rounding.

According to information provided by HHS, of the 43 activities for which PPHF allocations were made for fiscal years 2010 and 2011, about half (23 activities accounting for 72 percent of total fiscal year 2010 and 2011 allocations) received funding from regular (that is, non-PPHF) appropriations;[16] the remainder (20 activities accounting for 28 percent of total fiscal year 2010 and 2011 allocations) were funded solely from the PPHF during those 2 fiscal years. In fiscal year 2010, the three activities for which the largest PPHF allocations were made were:

---

[16]According to HHS, these 23 activities also received funding from HHS's regular appropriations in fiscal year 2010, 2011, or both. We use the term "regular appropriations" to refer to funding that is a product of the annual budget and appropriations process.

- HRSA's Primary Care Training and Enhancement ($198.1 million),

- CDC's National Public Health Improvement Initiative[17] ($50.0 million), and

- CDC's ARRA: Communities Putting Prevention to Work ($36.4 million).

In fiscal year 2011, the three activities for which the largest PPHF allocations were made were funded by CDC:

- Community Transformation Grants program ($146.3 million),

- Section 317 Immunization program ($100.0 million), and

- Coordinated Chronic Disease Prevention program ($51.7 million).

Activities for which the largest allocations were made in the three other HHS agencies during this 2-year period included AHRQ's support of the U.S. Preventive Services Task Force, SAMHSA's Primary and Behavioral Health Care Integration, and OS's Obesity Media Activities (see table 2).

---

[17]According to HHS officials, this activity was called Public Health Infrastructure in fiscal year 2010.

**Table 2: PPHF Allocations, by HHS Agency and Activity, Fiscal Years 2010 and 2011**

| Agency and activity | Fiscal year 2010 (in millions) | Fiscal year 2011 (in millions) | Total (in millions) |
|---|---|---|---|
| **Centers for Disease Control and Prevention (CDC)** | | | |
| Community Transformation Grants Program | — | $146.3 | $146.3 |
| Section 317 Immunization Program[a] | — | 100.0 | 100.0 |
| National Public Health Improvement Initiative[b] | $50.0 | 40.2 | 90.2 |
| Tobacco Prevention (Media and Quitlines)[a] | 14.5 | 50.0 | 64.5 |
| Epidemiology and Laboratory Capacity Grants[a] | 20.0 | 40.0 | 60.0 |
| Coordinated Chronic Disease Prevention Program[a] | — | 51.7 | 51.7 |
| CDC Healthcare Surveillance and Statistics[a] | 19.9 | 30.0 | 49.9 |
| ARRA: Communities Putting Prevention to Work | 36.4 | — | 36.4 |
| Environmental Public Health Tracking[a] | — | 35.0 | 35.0 |
| Public Health Workforce[a] | 7.5 | 25.0 | 32.5 |
| HIV/AIDS[a] | 30.4 | — | 30.4 |
| Racial and Ethnic Approaches to Community Health (REACH)[a] | — | 25.0 | 25.0 |
| Public Health Research[a] | — | 20.0 | 20.0 |
| Community Guide/Community Preventive Services Task Force[a] | 5.0 | 7.0 | 12.0 |
| Healthcare-Associated Infections[a] | — | 11.8 | 11.8 |
| Prevention Research Centers[a] | — | 10.0 | 10.0 |
| Workplace Wellness | — | 9.3 | 9.3 |
| National Youth Fitness Survey | — | 6.0 | 6.0 |
| ARRA: Evaluation | 4.0 | — | 4.0 |
| ARRA: Media | 4.0 | — | 4.0 |
| Education and Outreach Campaign Regarding Preventive Benefits | — | 2.0 | 2.0 |
| National Prevention Strategy | 0.1 | 1.0 | 1.1 |
| Promoting Obesity Prevention in Early Childhood Programs | — | 0.7 | 0.7 |
| Agency subtotal | 191.8 | 610.9 | 802.7 |
| **Health Resources and Services Administration (HRSA)** | | | |
| Primary Care Training and Enhancement[a] | 198.1 | — | 198.1 |
| Public Health Workforce Development[a] | 14.8 | 20.0 | 34.8 |
| Advanced Nursing Education[a] | 31.4 | — | 31.4 |
| Nurse Managed Care Centers | 15.3 | — | 15.3 |
| State Health Workforce Development Grants for Primary Care | 5.8 | — | 5.8 |
| HRSA Healthy Weight Collaborative and Activities | 5.0 | — | 5.0 |
| Nutrition, Physical Activity, and Screen Time Standards in Child Care Settings[a] | 0.3 | — | 0.3 |
| Agency subtotal | 270.7 | 20.0 | 290.7 |

| Agency and activity | Fiscal year 2010 (in millions) | Fiscal year 2011 (in millions) | Total (in millions) |
|---|---|---|---|
| **Substance Abuse and Mental Health Services Administration (SAMHSA)** | | | |
| Primary and Behavioral Health Care Integration[a] | 20.0 | 35.0 | 55.0 |
| Screening, Brief Intervention and Referral to Treatment[a] | — | 25.0 | 25.0 |
| SAMHSA Health Surveillance[a] | — | 18.0 | 18.0 |
| Suicide Prevention[a] | — | 10.0 | 10.0 |
| Agency subtotal | 20.0 | 88.0 | 108.0 |
| **Office of the Secretary (OS)** | | | |
| Obesity Media Activities | 9.1 | 9.1 | 18.2 |
| Tobacco Prevention Media | — | 10.0 | 10.0 |
| National Prevention, Health Promotion, and Public Health Council Planning | 1.0 | — | 1.0 |
| President's Council on Fitness, Sports, and Nutrition[a] | 0.9 | — | 0.9 |
| Tobacco Cessation | 0.9 | — | 0.9 |
| Healthy Living Innovations Awards | 0.1 | — | 0.1 |
| Agency subtotal | 12.0 | 19.1 | 31.1 |
| **Agency for Healthcare Research and Quality (AHRQ)** | | | |
| Clinical Preventive Services Task Force[a] | 5.0 | 7.0 | 12.0 |
| Clinical Preventive Services Research | — | 5.0 | 5.0 |
| Healthy Weight Practice-Based Research Networks | 0.5 | — | 0.5 |
| Agency subtotal | 5.5 | 12.0 | 17.5 |
| **Total PPHF allocations for all activities** | **$500.0** | **$750.0** | **$1,250.0** |

Source: GAO analysis of HHS information.

Notes: Total reported allocations from the PPHF in this table may not match—for example, they may be higher than—the total amounts awarded in grants or contracts (reported obligations) for each agency or activity. According to HHS officials, to carry out an activity, an agency may incur administrative expenses, including an agency's internal costs associated with managing and overseeing grants and contracts, not reflected in award amounts. Further, to the extent that an appropriation has not identified a particular amount for a specific activity, an agency may reallocate unobligated funds from that activity to another during the course of a fiscal year.

[a]In addition to PPHF funding, these 23 activities also received funding from regular appropriations. We use the term "regular appropriations" to refer to funding that is a product of the annual budget and appropriations process.

[b]According to HHS officials, this activity was called Public Health Infrastructure in fiscal year 2010.

For the 43 activities for which HHS allocated PPHF funds for fiscal years 2010 and 2011, HHS agencies awarded grants and contracts, and entered into interagency agreements, with the majority of funding awarded through grants (see table 3).[18] The number of award recipients for each activity ranged from 1 contractor for the AHRQ Healthy Weight Practice-Based Research Networks to 110 grantees receiving PPHF funding under HRSA's Primary Care Training and Enhancement activity. Recipients of PPHF funds were located in all 50 states, the District of Columbia, and 8 U.S. territories. (See apps. I-V for listings of recipients of PPHF funds and their locations.)

**Table 3: PPHF-Funded Awards by Funding Mechanism, Fiscal Years 2010 and 2011**

| | Fiscal year 2010 | | Fiscal year 2011 | |
|---|---|---|---|---|
| Funding mechanism | Number of awards | Amount awarded (in millions) | Number of awards | Amount awarded (in millions) |
| Grants | 545 | $416 | 663 | $463 |
| Contracts | 66 | 52 | 154 | 223 |
| Interagency agreements | 14 | 20 | 29 | 41 |
| **Total** | **625** | **$488** | **846** | **$727** |

Source: GAO analysis of HHS information.

Notes: This table presents the total amounts of PPHF funding awarded (reported as obligations) by HHS agencies through grants, contracts, and interagency agreements for fiscal years 2010 and 2011. Total amounts awarded (reported obligations) in this table may not match—for example, they may be lower than—the total amounts allocated for each fiscal year. According to HHS officials, to carry out an activity, an agency may incur administrative expenses, including an agency's internal costs associated with managing and overseeing grants and contracts, not reflected in award amounts. Further, to the extent that an appropriation has not identified a particular amount for a specific activity, an agency may reallocate unobligated funds from that activity to another during the course of a fiscal year.

PPHF-funded grants were awarded to state and local governments, tribal organizations, academic institutions, as well as national organizations and hospitals; eligibility for these awards was often limited to a certain type or types of entity. Our review of 58 funding opportunity announcements for PPHF-funded grants for fiscal years 2010 and 2011 found that state, local, territory, or tribal governments were eligible for the most grant opportunities in those years. While many funding opportunity

---

[18]Total amounts awarded (reported obligations) may not match—for example, they may be lower than—the total amounts allocated from the PPHF for each fiscal year. According to HHS, to carry out an activity, an agency may incur administrative expenses, including an agency's internal costs associated with managing and overseeing grants and contracts, not reflected in award amounts. Further, to the extent that an appropriation has not identified a particular amount for a specific activity, an agency may reallocate unobligated funds from that activity to another during the course of a fiscal year.

GAO-12-788 Prevention and Public Health Fund

announcements limited eligibility to one type of entity, others—including the funding opportunity announcement for the Community Transformation Grants program—listed multiple types of entities as eligible to apply for the PPHF-funded grants (see table 4).

**Table 4: Types of Entities Eligible for PPHF-Funded Grants Awarded in Fiscal Years 2010 and 2011**

| Type of entity | Fiscal year 2010 | | Fiscal year 2011 | | Total | |
|---|---|---|---|---|---|---|
| | Number of funding opportunities | Amount awarded (in millions) | Number of funding opportunities | Amount awarded (in millions) | Number of funding opportunities | Amount awarded (in millions) |
| Limited to state, local, territory, or tribal governments[a] | 13 | $125 | 13 | $228 | 26 | $353 |
| Limited to academic institutions or physician training programs[b] | 4 | 243 | 5 | 41 | 9 | 285 |
| Limited to national organizations[c] | 2 | 8 | 6 | 15 | 8 | 23 |
| Not limited to one type of recipient[d] | 5 | 40 | 8 | 168 | 11[e] | 208 |
| Other[f] | 0 | 0 | 4 | 10 | 4 | 10 |
| **Total** | **24** | **$416** | **36** | **$463** | **58[e]** | **$879** |

Source: GAO analysis of HHS information.

Note: This table presents information on the types of entities eligible to receive PPHF funded grants in fiscal years 2010 and 2011, including the total amounts of PPHF funding awarded (reported as obligated) by HHS agencies as a result of grants for fiscal years 2010 and 2011. Rows and columns may not total due to rounding.

[a]Includes grant funding opportunities that were limited to state, local, tribal, or territorial governments, or their bona fide agents, as well as tribal organizations and state partnerships such as a state workforce investment board.

[b]Includes grant funding opportunities that were limited to private and public educational institutions, as well as hospitals and other organizations that train providers.

[c]Includes grant funding opportunities that were limited to national, nonprofit, and public health organizations.

[d]Includes grant funding opportunities that were not limited to one type of entity—for example, multiple types of entities, including state, local, or tribal governments as well as nonprofit organizations were eligible to apply.

[e]Two funding announcements supported projects in both fiscal years 2010 and 2011. We examined 58 unique funding announcements.

[f]Includes funding opportunities limited to other types of organizations—for example, one that was limited to prevention epicenters and one that was limited to publicly funded community mental health and other community-based behavioral health agencies.

As reported by HHS, most PPHF-funded grants for fiscal years 2010 and 2011 were new grants, followed by supplemental and continuation grants (see table 5).

**Table 5: Number of Funding Opportunity Announcements and PPHF-Funded Grants, by Type of Grant, Fiscal Years 2010 and 2011**

| Type of grant in funding opportunity announcement[a] | Fiscal year 2010 | | Fiscal year 2011 | |
|---|---|---|---|---|
| | Number of funding opportunities | Number of grants | Number of funding opportunities | Number of grants |
| New | 17 | 419 | 17 | 202 |
| Supplemental | 7 | 126 | 11 | 218 |
| Continuation | 0 | 0 | 10 | 243 |
| **Total** | **24** | **545** | **36**[b] | **663** |

Source: GAO analysis of HHS funding opportunity announcements.

Note: This table presents the types of PPHF funded grants based on a review of 58 funding opportunity announcements identified by HHS for fiscal years 2010 and 2011. Two funding announcements supported projects in both fiscal years 2010 and 2011.

[a]A new grant provides funding for a project that is not currently receiving financial support, a continuation grant provides additional funding for one or more budget periods to a project for which financial support would otherwise end, and a supplemental grant increases funding for an approved project during a current budget period.

[b]The number of funding opportunities for each type do not sum to the column total because two funding announcements were used to make both new and continuation awards in fiscal year 2011. We examined 58 unique funding announcements.

HHS has not published a comprehensive list of agencies and activities for which PPHF funding was allocated and has not published a comprehensive list of all of the entities receiving PPHF funding in fiscal years 2010 and 2011; PPACA did not require HHS to do so.[19] For PPHF funding in fiscal year 2012, HHS established a website to provide information on activities supported from the PPHF, in response to provisions in the Consolidated Appropriations Act, 2012.[20] According to HHS officials, HHS does not plan to include information on activities

---

[19]Some information on activities and award recipients was reported in numerous press releases about activities funded by the PPHF in fiscal years 2010 and 2011 and on HHS and agency websites. For example, HHS issued press releases announcing some PPHF-funded awards with hyperlinks listing projects funded by the PPHF. In addition, a HHS website shows PPHF funding amounts by state and type of effort, such as community prevention, clinical prevention, or research and data collection. See http://www.healthcare.gov/news/factsheets/2011/02/prevention02092011a.html (accessed Aug. 6, 2012).

[20]According to HHS, this website will provide information on the fiscal year 2012 planned allocation of PPHF funds, funding opportunities, and the recipients of awards, with information to be posted as it becomes available. See http://www.hhs.gov/open/recordsandreports/prevention/ (accessed June 12, 2012).

funded in fiscal years 2010 and 2011 on this website, and as of May 2012, was still evaluating how it will use the website in fiscal year 2013.

## Process and Criteria for Allocating and Awarding PPHF Funds for Fiscal Years 2010 and 2011

HHS implemented an abbreviated process to allocate PPHF funds for fiscal years 2010 and 2011 because of the timing when PPACA was enacted, according to HHS. PPACA was signed into law on March 23, 2010, 1 week before the midpoint of fiscal year 2010 and over a month after the President had released his fiscal year 2011 budget request. (See fig. 2 for a timeline of key events.)

**Figure 2: PPHF Key Event Timeline, Fiscal Years 2010 and 2011**

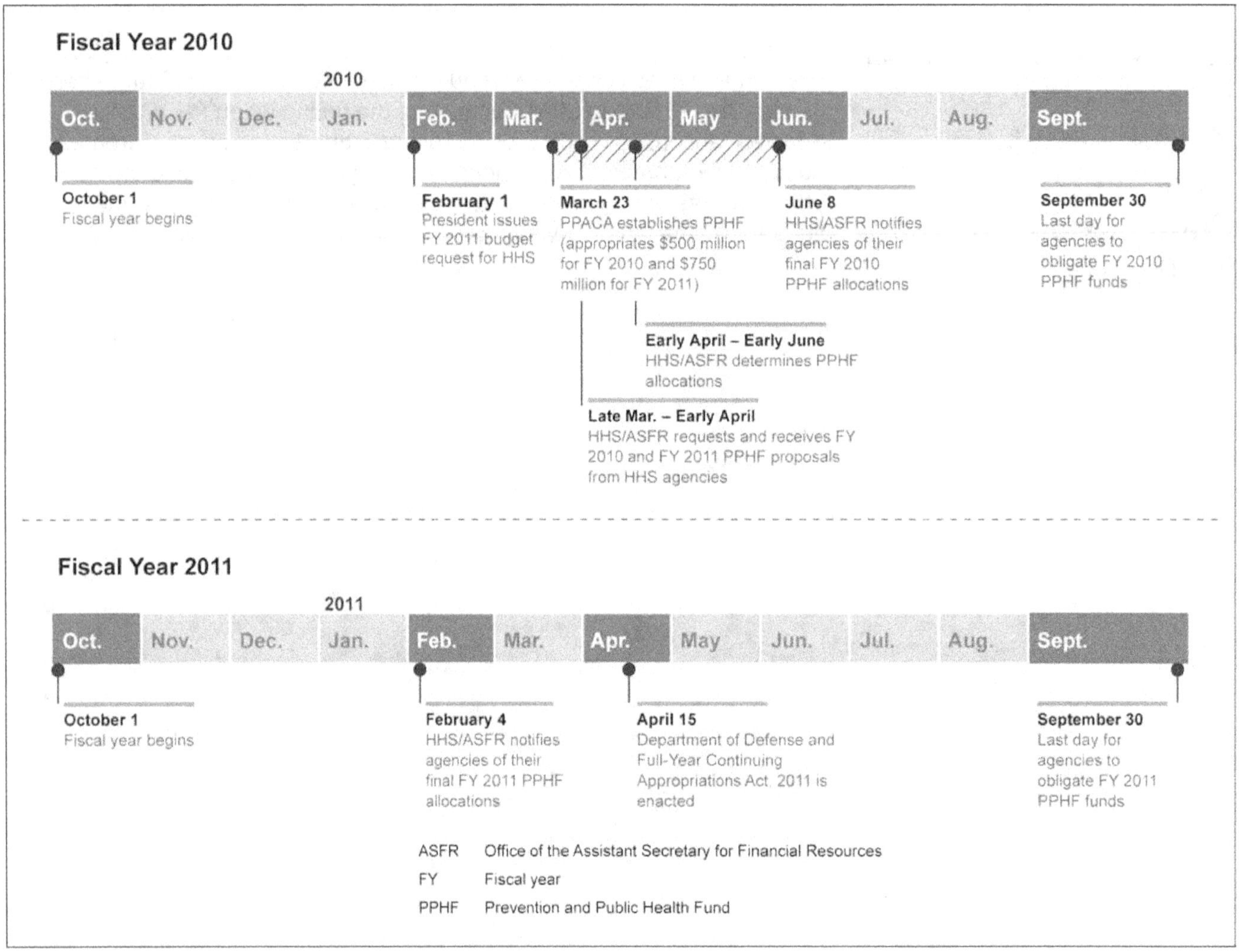

## Fiscal Year 2010

2010

| Oct. | Nov. | Dec. | Jan. | Feb. | Mar. | Apr. | May | Jun. | Jul. | Aug. | Sept. |

**October 1**
Fiscal year begins

**February 1**
President issues FY 2011 budget request for HHS

**March 23**
PPACA establishes PPHF (appropriates $500 million for FY 2010 and $750 million for FY 2011)

**June 8**
HHS/ASFR notifies agencies of their final FY 2010 PPHF allocations

**September 30**
Last day for agencies to obligate FY 2010 PPHF funds

**Early April – Early June**
HHS/ASFR determines PPHF allocations

**Late Mar. – Early April**
HHS/ASFR requests and receives FY 2010 and FY 2011 PPHF proposals from HHS agencies

## Fiscal Year 2011

2011

| Oct. | Nov. | Dec. | Jan. | Feb. | Mar. | Apr. | May | Jun. | Jul. | Aug. | Sept. |

**October 1**
Fiscal year begins

**February 4**
HHS/ASFR notifies agencies of their final FY 2011 PPHF allocations

**April 15**
Department of Defense and Full-Year Continuing Appropriations Act, 2011 is enacted

**September 30**
Last day for agencies to obligate FY 2011 PPHF funds

ASFR    Office of the Assistant Secretary for Financial Resources
FY       Fiscal year
PPHF    Prevention and Public Health Fund

Source: GAO summary of HHS information.

HHS implemented an abbreviated process for allocating PPHF funds for fiscal years 2010 and 2011 due to the timing of PPACA in relation to the budget formulation process for those years.[21] That is, because the President's budget request, along with agency justifications, had already been submitted, HHS did not have the opportunity to lay out its plans for how PPHF funds would be spent for fiscal years 2010 and 2011. According to ASFR officials, for fiscal years 2012 and 2013 HHS considered which activities to support with PPHF funding through the annual budget formulation process.[22]

In its abbreviated process, HHS requested proposals for PPHF funding from agencies. HHS did not develop HHS-wide criteria for fiscal years 2010 and 2011; instead HHS instructed agencies to use activities cited in the PPACA provisions establishing the PPHF as guidance for developing proposals for activities for which HHS could allocate PPHF funding. According to HHS, the proposed activities were also aligned with existing departmental priorities. HHS then evaluated agency proposals and allocated and transferred PPHF funds to the corresponding appropriations accounts, guided in fiscal year 2011 by proposed legislative language. Agencies then evaluated applications and selected projects to fund with their available PPHF funds. Table 6 provides a description of actions taken in each step for allocating and awarding PPHF funds for fiscal years 2010 and 2011, as reported by HHS and agency officials.

---

[21]Federal agencies typically begin developing their budget requests in the spring (or earlier) each year, at least 9 months before the President submits his budget request to Congress, and about 17 months before the start of the fiscal year to which the budget requests pertains. For fiscal year 2010 that started on October 1, 2009, the President released his budget request in February 2009, and agencies would have begun work on their budgets in spring 2008. For fiscal year 2011, agencies would have begun work on their budgets in spring 2009. As part of this budget and appropriations process for regular appropriations, agencies prepare and submit materials (budget justifications) to accompany the President's budget that lay out their plans for how funds would be spent. Because of the timing of PPACA, HHS did not have the opportunity to include PPHF funds in its submissions for fiscal years 2010 and 2011.

[22]HHS's congressional budget justifications for fiscal years 2012 and 2013 identified the activities for which HHS proposed allocating PPHF funds in those years. According to HHS, the department's annual budget formulation process includes participation of the Secretary's Budget Council, which consists of the HHS Deputy Secretary, the Secretary-appointed policy counselors, and other select leadership within the Office of the Secretary who advise the Secretary on departmental issues, including the annual HHS budget.

**Table 6: HHS Process for Allocating and Awarding PPHF Funds, Fiscal Years 2010 and 2011**

| Step | HHS/Agency action |
|------|-------------------|
| 1. Agencies develop PPHF proposals | In late March to early April 2010, HHS requested agencies to submit proposals for fiscal years 2010 and 2011 PPHF funding. HHS officials reported that the shortened time frames did not allow for development of HHS-wide written criteria for developing PPHF proposals. In lieu of HHS-wide criteria, agencies were referred to the activities cited in PPACA related to PPHF funding as guiding principles in developing agency proposals—specifically, that PPHF is "for programs authorized by the Public Health Service Act, for prevention, wellness, and public health activities including prevention research, health screenings, and initiatives, such as the Community Transformation grant program, the Education and Outreach Campaign Regarding Preventive Benefits, and immunization programs."[a] HHS also requested that agency proposals focus on existing programs or programs that could be implemented in a short time frame. For example: <br><br> • AHRQ officials reported using existing criteria for its Prevention and Care Management program, including improving primary care and clinical outcomes through health care redesign, clinical-community linkages, self-management support, integration of health information technology, and care coordination, to identify activities to propose for PPHF funding. <br><br> • SAMHSA officials reported proposing funding for additional grants under existing activities, including additional grants for suicide prevention. |
| 2. HHS allocates PPHF funds to agencies and activities | After receiving proposals from agencies for fiscal year 2010 PPHF funding, HHS officials allocated and provided for the transfer of funds so that funds could be obligated before the end of the fiscal year. For example, they did this by allocating PPHF funds for activities that had existing mechanisms in place for implementation. In fiscal year 2010, HHS made the largest PPHF allocation for HRSA's Primary Care Training and Enhancement activity as part of an initiative to increase the nation's supply of primary care providers. <br><br> According to HHS officials, for allocation decisions for both fiscal years 2010 and 2011, HHS leadership, including members of the Secretary's Budget Council,[b] reviewed and evaluated PPHF proposals, and developed final allocations. For fiscal year 2011, HHS also used proposed legislative language as guidance for allocating PPHF funds. |
| 3. Agencies select PPHF projects for funding | In general, each agency administering activities for which PPHF allocations and transfers were made issued funding announcements and many agencies reported using their regular review process to select project applications for PPHF funding. Agencies also reported using existing criteria—and in some cases language from PPACA as additional criteria—to select grants and contracts. For example: <br><br> • AHRQ officials reported that fiscal year 2010 and 2011 PPHF-funded grants and contracts, as well as non-PPHF awards, were competitively selected based on peer reviews and scoring. <br><br> • CDC officials reported that the specific criteria used to evaluate proposals were tailored to each funding announcement—common rating criteria included demonstration of public health need; feasibility and effectiveness of activities, staffing plan, and budget; defined, measurable, and achievable goals; and efficient and effective use of resources. CDC officials reported that they also used language from PPACA as criteria for rating applications for PPHF funds for fiscal years 2010 and 2011. <br><br> • HRSA officials told us that they generally invest funding (including PPHF funds) in programs that have the potential of having a national impact. According to HRSA, individual projects, or grants, are selected using a competitive process, are independently reviewed, and generally reflect geographic distribution. |

Source: GAO summary of HHS information.

[a]Because CDC refers to the "Community Transformation Grants program", we use that name in referring to the program in this report.

[b]The Secretary's Budget Council consists of the HHS Deputy Secretary, the Secretary-appointed policy counselors, and other select leadership within the Office of the Secretary who advise the Secretary on departmental issues, including the annual HHS budget.

As part of the abbreviated process HHS used for fiscal years 2010 and 2011, following the enactment of PPACA, HHS developed a PPHF allocation plan then consulted with staff from the authorizing and appropriations committees prior to transferring the funds. Specifically, HHS told us that prior to transferring PPHF funds within HHS for fiscal years 2010 and 2011, officials notified minority and majority staff from authorizing and appropriations committees including: the House Appropriations Subcommittee on Labor, Health and Human Services, Education, and Related Agencies; the Senate Appropriations Subcommittee on Labor, Health and Human Services, Education, and Related Agencies; the House Energy and Commerce Committee; and, the Senate Committee on Health, Education, Labor and Pensions. In addition, for fiscal year 2011, HHS told us that the department used language for the proposed allocation in the fiscal year HHS appropriation[23] as a guide for allocating the $750 million available from the PPHF that year. HHS also reported consulting with the authorizing and appropriations committees prior to executing the transfer of funds for the fiscal year 2011 allocation.

For fiscal years 2010 and 2011, HHS did not formally solicit input from outside stakeholders on the PPHF allocation process, according to HHS officials. But HHS officials reported that a wide range of stakeholders, including states, nonprofit organizations, community-based organizations, and coalitions, proactively provided HHS and agencies with input on the use of PPHF funds, which was considered by HHS leadership during the decision-making process.

---

[23]156 Cong. Rec. S9026 (daily ed. Dec. 14, 2010) (section 4 of proposed S. Amdt. 4805 to H. R. 3082 provided that the explanatory statement by the Chairman of the Senate Committee on Appropriations, which specified amounts to be transferred from the PPHF to HHS agencies for specific activities administered by those agencies, was to have the same effect with respect to the allocation of funds as if it were a joint explanatory statement of a committee of conference) (the amendment was not agreed to and the proposed language did not become law); 156 Cong. Rec. S9799 (explanatory statement by the Chairman of the Senate Committee on Appropriations for proposed fiscal year 2011 HHS appropriation); S9849 (daily ed. Dec. 14, 2010 (portion of explanatory statement providing for transfers from the PPHF)).

## HHS Reporting of Performance Measures, Targets, and Outcomes of Activities and Projects Receiving PPHF Funding

HHS has relied on its agencies to establish performance measures and targets and to track outcomes of PPHF activities. For the 23 activities for which PPHF allocations were made and that received funding through regular appropriations, performance measures, targets, and outcomes data were generally not specific to PPHF-funded projects, but applied to the entire activity regardless of the funding source. For example, SAMHSA used both regular appropriations and PPHF funds for existing activities, such as suicide prevention. Moreover, SAMHSA evaluates the performance of the suicide prevention activities as a whole and does not have separate performance measures for the PPHF-funded projects. For individual projects receiving PPHF funding, performance measures were frequently established in funding opportunity announcements.

HHS agency officials told us that it is too early to report outcomes for many activities for which PPHF funding was allocated because many projects receiving PPHF funding in fiscal year 2010, 2011, or both are multiyear projects or have not yet completed project evaluations, and outcomes have not been measured or reported.[24] For example, one performance measure of HRSA's Primary Care Training and Enhancement activity—an activity that received PPHF funding in fiscal year 2010—is the number of primary care physicians supported with PPHF funding who complete their education; however, while data on the number of individuals training to be physicians who are supported with PPHF funding are available, outcome data on the numbers completing their programs will not be available until fiscal year 2014, the year the first cohort of physicians supported by fiscal year 2010 PPHF funding will finish their training. Table 7 presents information on performance measures and available information on targets and outcomes for the three HHS activities for which the largest PPHF allocations were made for fiscal years 2010 and 2011. Collectively, HHS allocated a total of $198.1 million for fiscal year 2010 and $246.3 million for fiscal year 2011 for these three activities.

---

[24]Agency officials said that some performance measures and outcomes for activities receiving PPHF funding will be reported as part of their agencies' routine Government Performance and Results Act (GPRA) performance reporting. Pub. L. No. 103-62, 107 Stat. 285 (1993). GPRA, which was recently amended by the GPRA Modernization Act of 2010, requires agencies to establish outcome-oriented goals and performance indicators to measure overall progress toward these goals. *See* Pub. L. No. 111-352, 124 Stat. 3866 (2011); GAO, *Managing for Results: Opportunities for Congress to Address Government Performance Issues,* GAO-12-215R (Washington, D.C.: Dec. 9, 2011).

GAO-12-788 Prevention and Public Health Fund

**Table 7: Overall Performance Measures, Targets, and Outcome Information for the Three Activities for Which HHS Allocated the Most PPHF Funding, Fiscal Years 2010 and 2011**

| Activity (agency) and PPHF allocation amounts | Performance measures, targets, and outcomes[a] |
|---|---|
| Primary Care Training and Enhancement (HRSA)<br><br>Fiscal year 2010: $198.1 million | Under this activity, which includes HRSA's Expansion of Physician Assistant Training program and Primary Care Residency Expansion program, HRSA performance measures and targets include the following:<br><br>• Number of physician assistants who complete their education supported by PPHF funding. (Target of 140 for fiscal year 2012.)<br><br>• Number of primary care physicians who complete their education supported by PPHF funding. (Target of 172 for fiscal year 2014.)<br><br>According to HRSA, outcome data for these performance measure are not yet available, because students initially funded with PPHF funding in fiscal year 2010 will complete their training programs in fiscal years 2012 (physician assistants) and 2014 (physicians). |
| Community Transformation Grants Program (CDC)<br><br>Fiscal year 2011: $146.3 million | As of May 14, 2012, CDC had not finalized performance measures or targets for this activity. CDC's draft performance measures, for which CDC estimated that targets will be available around October 2012, include the following:<br><br>• Number of people with increased access to smoke-free or tobacco-free environments in settings such as workplaces, restaurants, campuses, and outdoor places.<br><br>• Number of people with increased access to environments with healthy food or beverage options, including in schools, workplaces, and other community settings.<br><br>• Number of people with increased access to physical activity opportunities, including in schools, workplaces, and other community settings.<br><br>• Number of people with increased access to systems that support control of high blood pressure and of high cholesterol in health care and other community settings.<br><br>CDC had not reported data on outcomes as of May 2012. |
| Section 317 Immunization Program (CDC)<br><br>Fiscal year 2011: $100.0 million | To ensure that children and adolescents are appropriately vaccinated, CDC performance measures and targets for this activity include the following:[b]<br><br>• Sustain immunization coverage in children 19-35 months of age for one dose of measles, mumps, and rubella vaccine. (Target of at least 90 percent for fiscal year 2011.)<br><br>• Achieve immunization coverage of at least 90 percent in children 19-35 months of age for at least four doses of pneumococcal conjugate vaccine. (Target of at least 87 percent for fiscal year 2011.)<br><br>• Achieve immunization coverage of at least 60 percent in children 19-35 months of age for two to three doses of rotavirus vaccine. (Target of at least 52 percent for fiscal year 2011.)<br><br>• Achieve or sustain immunization coverage of at least 70 percent in adolescents 13 to 15 years of age for one dose Tdap (tetanus and diphtheria toxoids and acellular pertussis). (Target of at least 67 percent for fiscal year 2011.)<br><br>• Achieve or sustain immunization coverage of at least 70 percent in adolescents 13 to 15 years of age for one dose meningococcal conjugate vaccine. (Target of at least 66 percent for fiscal year 2011.)<br><br>According to CDC, data on outcomes for fiscal year 2011 will be available by September 30, 2012. |

Source: GAO analysis of HRSA and CDC information.

<sup></sup>ᵃSome of these targets are consistent with objectives in Health People 2020, which provides a comprehensive set of 10-year national goals and objectives for improving the health of all Americans. For example, Health People 2020 includes objectives to "increase tobacco-free environments in schools" and to "achieve and maintain effective vaccination coverage levels for universally recommended vaccines among young children." For more information, see http://www.healthypeople.gov/2020/about/default.aspx.

ᵇAccording to CDC, the targets reflect the impact of funding from both regular appropriations and PPHF funds.

As of July 2012, information was available on some projects receiving PPHF funding in fiscal years 2010 and 2011—for example, CDC posted information on activities planned by individual projects funded by its Community Transformation Grants program, which was initiated in late fiscal year 2011.[25] At the same time, however, information on all fiscal year 2010 and 2011 outcomes was not reported.[26]

## Agency Comments

HHS reviewed a draft of this report and provided technical comments, which we incorporated as appropriate.

As arranged with your offices, unless you publicly announce its contents earlier, we plan no further distribution of this report until 30 days after its issue date. At that time, we will send copies of this report to the Secretary of Health and Human Services and interested congressional committees. In addition, the report will be available at no charge on the GAO website at http://www.gao.gov.

---

[25]See http://www.cdc.gov/communitytransformation/index.htm (accessed July 23, 2012).

[26]For fiscal year 2012, HHS is required to report on PPHF-funded projects valued at $25,000 or more. The Consolidated Appropriations Act, 2012 requires HHS to post on its website semiannual reports summarizing the activities undertaken for each PPHF-funded grant or contract of $25,000 or more (to be posted no later than 30 days after the end of each 6-month period). Pub. L. No. 112-74, § 220, 125 Stat. 1085-1086. As of July 23, 2012, no semiannual reports had been posted on the website. See http://www.hhs.gov/open/recordsandreports/prevention/ (accessed July 23, 2012).

If you or your staff have any questions regarding this report, please contact me at (202) 512-7114 or iritanik@gao.gov. Contact points for our Office of Congressional Relations and Public Affairs may be found on the last page of this report. GAO staff who made key contributions to this report are listed in appendix VI.

Katherine Iritani
Director, Health Care

# Appendix I: Agency for Healthcare Research and Quality—Prevention and Public Health Fund Awards by Activity

This appendix presents information on awards made by the Agency for Healthcare Research and Quality (AHRQ) for Prevention and Public Health Fund (PPHF) activities with funds allocated and transferred from the PPHF for fiscal years (FY) 2010 and 2011. For each AHRQ activity that received PPHF funding, tables 8 through 12 summarize information on awards made with those funds through grants and contracts for each fiscal year.[1] Award information was provided by the Department of Health and Human Services' (HHS) Assistant Secretary for Financial Resources, AHRQ, or reported in the funding opportunity announcements (FOA) HHS identified as being associated with the activity and awards.

The information presented in this appendix, including the purpose of the PPHF-funded activity, was obtained from HHS. Due to the large number of awards, we did not edit the award recipient information to correct typographical or grammatical errors, or clarify the information provided. In general, we reprinted the abbreviations and acronyms provided by HHS and the legislative authority cited in the FOA or otherwise provided by HHS. We did not independently verify the legislative authority. Totals in this appendix (reported obligations) may not match—for example, they may be lower than—the amounts in table 2 (reported allocations). According to HHS officials, to carry out an activity, an agency may incur administrative expenses, including an agency's internal costs associated with managing and overseeing grants and contracts, not reflected in award amounts. Further, to the extent that an appropriation has not identified a particular amount for a specific activity, an agency may reallocate unobligated funds from that activity to another during the course of a fiscal year.

**Activity**: Clinical Preventive Services Task Force

The purpose of this activity is to support the U.S. Preventive Services Task Force (USPSTF), an independent panel of private-sector experts in prevention and primary care, including support for a Scientific Resource Center, a preventive medicine residency rotation program, staff support, and to develop and finalize updated evidence reports.

---

[1]The tables present information on cooperative agreements with grants, and include information on interagency agreements with contracts.

GAO-12-788 Prevention and Public Health Fund

- **Fiscal year 2010**: $5.0 million (2 contracts)

- **Fiscal year 2011**: $6.8 million (2 contracts)

**Table 8: FY 2010 Contracts, Clinical Preventive Services Task Force**

| Recipient | Purpose | State | Award (dollars) |
|---|---|---|---|
| ABT Associates, Inc. | Specialized Communications for USPSTF | MA | $4,000,000 |
| Oregon Evidence-based Practice Center (EPC) for USPSTF Reviews | USPSTF Reviews | OR | 1,010,937 |
| **Total (2 awards)** | | | **$5,010,937** |

Source: GAO analysis of HHS information.

**Table 9: FY 2011 Contracts, Clinical Preventive Services Task Force**

| Recipient | Purpose | State | Award (dollars) |
|---|---|---|---|
| ABT Associates, Inc. | Specialized Communications for USPSTF | MA | $3,776,974 |
| Oregon Evidence-based Practice Center (EPC) for USPSTF Reviews | USPSTF Reviews | OR | 3,000,000 |
| **Total (2 awards)** | | | **$6,776,974** |

Source: GAO analysis of HHS information.

## Activity: Clinical Preventive Services Research

The purpose of this activity is to support integrated, multiproject research programs that will work with a well-defined, central research focus to contribute to addressing the research and implementation gaps identified as part of the development of the HHS National Prevention and National Quality Strategies.

- **Fiscal year 2010**: None

- **Fiscal year 2011**: $4.8 million (3 grants totaling $4.3 million and 1 contract for $0.5 million)

**Table 10: FY 2011 Grants, Clinical Preventive Services Research**

| Announcement | Recipient | State | Award (dollars) |
| --- | --- | --- | --- |
| Research Centers for Excellence in Clinical Preventive Services (RFA-HS-11-005) | University of North Carolina, Chapel Hill | NC | $1,500,000 |
| | University of Colorado, Denver | CO | 1,483,338 |
| | Northwestern University | IL | 1,365,757 |
| **Purpose (award type)**: To support Research Centers for Excellence in Clinical Preventive Services to conduct research and development activities in order to generate new knowledge and develop tools and resources to improve health and health care through clinical preventive services. Core infrastructure should include: training, education, and robust dissemination capabilities, and may, in addition, focus on the provision of specific methodologic support to the Center. Each Research Center application must propose a body of work addressing one of three programmatic areas: (1) patient safety; (2) health equity; or, (3) health care system implementation. (New) | **Total (3 awards)** | | **$4,349,095** |
| **Legislative Authority**: 42 U.S.C. 299a(a), which authorizes AHRQ to conduct and support research, support demonstration projects, and disseminate information on health care and on systems for the delivery of such care, including activities with respect to clinical practice, including primary care and practice-oriented research. See 42 U.S.C. 299a(a)4. | | | |
| **Eligibility**: Public or non-profit private institution, such as a university, college, or a faith-based or community-based organization; Units of local or State government; Eligible agencies of the Federal government; Indian/Native American Tribal Government (Federally Recognized); Indian/Native American Tribal Government (Other than Federally Recognized); and Indian/Native American Tribally Designated Organizations. | | | |

Source: GAO analysis of HHS information.

**Table 11: FY 2011 Contract, Clinical Preventive Services Research**

| Recipient | Purpose | State | Award (dollars) |
|---|---|---|---|
| Abt Associates, Inc. | Technical assistance and evaluation of grant program. | MD | $484,986 |
| **Total (1 award)** | | | **$484,986** |

Source: GAO analysis of HHS information.

## Activity: Healthy Weight Practice-Based Research Networks

The purpose of this activity is to promote innovative efforts to improve the management of obese patients in primary care by (1) supporting the development and evaluation of scalable and sustainable linkages between primary care practices and community-based resources to support obesity treatment and management across the lifespan; and (2) creating an implementation guide on obesity management to be disseminated widely to diverse primary care settings that describes optimal processes for developing, assessing, and maintaining effective linkages with community-based programs.

- **Fiscal year 2010**: $0.5 million (1 contract)

- **Fiscal year 2011**: None

**Table 12: FY 2010 Contract, Healthy Weight Practice-Based Research Networks**

| Recipient | Purpose | State | Award (dollars) |
|---|---|---|---|
| Colorado Practice-based Research Network (PBRN) Healthy Weight | To create a guide for primary care practices to build linkages with community based organizations in support of healthy weight programs. | CO | $489,063 |
| **Total (1 award)** | | | **$489,063** |

Source: GAO analysis of HHS information.

# Appendix II: Centers for Disease Control and Prevention—Prevention and Public Health Fund Awards by Activity

This appendix presents information on awards made by the Centers for Disease Control and Prevention (CDC) for Prevention and Public Health Fund (PPHF) activities with funds allocated and transferred from the PPHF for fiscal years (FY) 2010 and 2011. For each CDC activity that received PPHF funding, tables 13 through 62 summarize information on awards made with those funds through grants and contracts for each fiscal year.[1] Award information was provided by HHS's Assistant Secretary for Financial Resources, CDC, or reported in the funding opportunity announcements (FOA) HHS identified as being associated with the activity and awards.

The information presented in this appendix, including the purpose of the PPHF-funded activity, was obtained from HHS. Due to the large number of awards, we did not edit the award recipient information to correct typographical or grammatical errors, or clarify the information provided. In general, we reprinted the abbreviations and acronyms provided by HHS and the legislative authority cited in the FOA or otherwise provided by HHS. We did not independently verify the legislative authority. Totals in this appendix (reported obligations) may not match—for example, they may be lower than—the amounts in table 2 (reported allocations). According to HHS officials, to carry out an activity, an agency may incur administrative expenses, including an agency's internal costs associated with managing and overseeing grants and contracts, not reflected in award amounts. Further, to the extent that an appropriation has not identified a particular amount for a specific activity, an agency may reallocate unobligated funds from that activity to another during the course of a fiscal year.

Activity: Community Transformation Grants Program

The purpose of this activity is to support community-level efforts to reduce chronic diseases such as heart disease, cancer, stroke, and diabetes. By promoting healthy lifestyles, especially among population groups experiencing the greatest burden of chronic disease, these funded projects are designed to help improve health, reduce health disparities, and control health care spending.

---

[1]The tables present information on cooperative agreements with grants, and include information on interagency agreements with contracts.

- **Fiscal year 2010**: None

- **Fiscal year 2011**: $139.3 million (68 grants in three funding
  announcements totaling $107.9 million and contracts totaling
  $31.4 million)

**Table 13: FY 2011 Grants, Community Transformation Grants Program**

| Announcements (3) | Recipient | State | Award (dollars) |
|---|---|---|---|
| 1. Public Prevention Health Fund: Community Transformation Grants (CDC-RFA-DP11-1103PPHF11)<br><br>**Purpose (award type)**: To create healthier communities by (1) building capacity to implement broad evidence and practice-based policy, environmental, programmatic and infrastructure changes, as appropriate, in large counties, and in states, tribes and territories, including in rural and frontier areas; and (2) supporting implementation of such interventions in five strategic areas (1) tobacco-free living, (2) active living and healthy eating, (3) high impact evidence-based clinical and other preventive services, (4) social and emotional wellness, and (5) healthy and safe physical environment. (New)<br><br>**Legislative Authority**: Sections 4002 and 4201 of the Affordable Care Act.<br><br>**Eligibility**: Limited to state and local governmental agencies, or their Bona Fide Agent or the equivalent, as well as, state and local nonprofit organizations, federally recognized American Indian Tribes and Alaska Native Villages, tribal organizations, and Urban Indian Health programs. | Texas State Dept of Health Services | TX | $10,000,000 |
| | Los Angeles County Health Services Dept | CA | 9,848,011 |
| | New York State Dept of Health | NY | 8,391,881 |
| | NC State Dept/Hlth & Human Services | NC | 7,466,092 |
| | Public Health Institute | CA | 5,926,365 |
| | Illinois State Dept of Public Health | IL | 4,781,121 |
| | University of Wisconsin-Madison | WI | 4,700,000 |
| | South Carolina State Dept of Hlth/Env | SC | 4,624,724 |
| | Minnesota State Dept of Health | MN | 3,603,724 |
| | Washington State Department of Health | WA | 3,256,347 |
| | Massachusetts State Dept of Pub Health | MA | 3,079,988 |
| | County/San Diego Health/Human Ser/Ag | CA | 3,053,793 |
| | Iowa State Dept of Public Health | IA | 3,007,856 |
| | Maryland State Dept of Hlth/Mtl Hygiene | MD | 1,945,289 |
| | WV State Dept Hlth/Human Rscs | WV | 1,883,603 |
| | Broward Regional Health Planning Council | FL | 1,766,476 |
| | City of Philadelphia Public Health Dept | PA | 1,547,297 |
| | New Mexico State Department of Health | NM | 1,500,000 |
| | Maine State Dept/Health/Human Servs | ME | 1,318,301 |
| | Hennepin County Health and Human Services | MN | 1,156,212 |
| | Austin Health and Human Services Department | TX | 1,026,158 |
| | San Francisco Dept of Public Health | CA | 815,358 |
| | South Dakota State Dept of Health | SD | 812,383 |
| | Tacoma-Pierce County Health Department | WA | 796,836 |
| | Montana State Dept/Pub Hlth & Human Srvs | MT | 769,195 |
| | University of Rochester | NY | 733,703 |
| | Louisville Metro Department of Health | KY | 721,594 |
| | OK City County Health Department | OK | 716,704 |
| | Mid-American Regional Council Comm. Services | MO | 705,708 |

| Announcements (3) | Recipient | State | Award (dollars) |
|---|---|---|---|
| | Vermont Department of Health | VT | 621,760 |
| | Denver Health and Hospital Authority | CO | 610,345 |
| | Douglas County Health Department | NE | 510,199 |
| | My Brother's Keeper | MS | 500,000 |
| | Sault St. Marie Tribe of Chippewa Indians | MI | 500,000 |
| | Houston City Health & Human Services | TX | 500,000 |
| | Operation Unite | KY | 500,000 |
| | Louisiana State Dept of Hlth & Hospitals | LA | 500,000 |
| | Austen Bioinnovation Institute In Akron | OH | 500,000 |
| | Toyiabe Indian Health Project | CA | 500,000 |
| | New Jersey State Dept/Health/Senior Srvs | NJ | 500,000 |
| | Great Lakes Inter-Tribal Council | WI | 499,982 |
| | Fresno County Department of Public Health | CA | 499,695 |
| | Southeast Alaska Reg Hlth Consortium | AK | 499,588 |
| | Fairfax County Neighborhood And Comm. Srvcs | VA | 499,559 |
| | Utah State Department of Health | UT | 499,366 |
| | Sierra Health Foundation | CA | 499,229 |
| | Cobb Public Health | GA | 499,000 |
| | Confederated Tribes of the Chehalis Reservation | WA | 498,663 |
| | Bernalillo County Office of Environmental Health | NM | 497,353 |
| | Connecticut State Dept of Public Health | CT | 493,891 |
| | Ventura County | CA | 481,036 |
| | County of Kern Public Health Services Dept | CA | 416,577 |
| | North Dakota State Department of Health | ND | 370,684 |
| | Spectrum Health Hospitals | MI | 333,321 |
| | Stanislaus County Health Services Agency | CA | 293,899 |
| | Lancaster General Health | PA | 233,577 |
| | Sophie Trettevick Indian Health Center | WA | 218,929 |
| | Yukon-Kuskokwim Health Corporation | AK | 193,340 |
| | Public Health - Dayton And Montgomery County | OH | 180,246 |
| | Ulkerreuil A. Klengar | PW | 147,106 |
| | **Total (60 awards)** | | **$103,552,064** |

| Announcements (3) | Recipient | State | Award (dollars) |
|---|---|---|---|
| 2. Public Prevention Health Fund: National Dissemination and Support for Community Transformation Grants (CDC-RFA-DP11-1115PPHF11)<br><br>**Purpose (award type):** To support the efforts of the Community Transformation Grants program (CDC-RFA-DP11-1103PPHF11) by funding national network(s) of community-based organizations. Also to support, disseminate and amplify successful program models and activities as prescribed under statutory authority [Section 4201 (c) (5) of ACA]. (New)<br><br>**Legislative Authority:** Sections 4002 and 4201 of the Patient Protection and Affordable Care Act (ACA).<br><br>**Eligibility:** National network(s) of community based organizations. | National Council of the Young Men's Christian Association | IL | $1,300,000 |
|  | National REACH Coalition | CA | 900,000 |
|  | American Lung Association | DC | 800,000 |
|  | Community Anti-Drug Coalitions of America | VA | 300,000 |
|  | American Public Health Association | DC | 300,000 |
|  | Occidental College | CA | 300,000 |
|  | Asian Pacific Partners for Empowerment, Advocacy and Leadership | CA | 300,000 |
|  | **Total (7 awards)** |  | **$4,200,000** |
| 3. Competitive Program Expansion Supplement for CDC-RFA-HM08-805: Strengthen and Improve the Nation's Capacity through National, Non-profit, Professional Public Health Organizations to Increase Health Protection and Health Equity (CDC-RFA-HM08-8050402PHFF11)<br><br>**Purpose (award type):** To support the provision of capacity building assistance to state, tribal, local and territorial health departments that ensures performance improvement and successful adoption of best or promising practices to address key areas of public health infrastructure investments. (Supplement)<br><br>**Legislative Authority:** Sections 301 and 317 of the Public Health Service Act (PHS Act), 42 USC, 241 and 247b as amended. Funding is appropriated under the Affordable Care Act (PL 111-148), Title IV, Section 4002 (Prevention and Public Health Fund).<br><br>**Eligibility:** Limited to specific national, non-profit, public health professional organizations funded through the competitive funding opportunity announcement CDC-RFA-HM08-805. | National Association of City/County Health Officials | DC | 140,000 |
|  | **Total (1 award)** |  | **$140,000** |

Source: GAO analysis of HHS information.

**Table 14: FY 2011 Contracts, Community Transformation Grants Program**

| Recipient | Purpose | State | Award (dollars) |
|---|---|---|---|
| ICF Macro, Inc | TA and Training Contract | GA | $6,035,730 |
| Research Triangle Institute | Community Transformation Grants – Evaluation Technical Assistance, Training Services, and Performance Monitoring | GA | 5,835,132 |
| FHI Development 360 LLC | Community Transformation Grants Program Evaluation – Enhanced Evaluation Techniques | GA | 5,396,166 |
| Four Seasons Environmental, Inc. | CDC Program Oversight & Implementation | GA | 4,430,683 |
| Research Triangle Institute | Social Media Contract | GA | 4,319,460 |
| ICF Macro, Inc | Modeling and Cost Benefit Analysis Contract | GA | 3,281,366 |
| Global Evaluation & Applied Research Solutions (GEARS) | Extramural Staffing Contract | GA | 678,033 |
| Deloitte Consulting, LLP | CDC Program Oversight & Implementation | GA | 477,725 |
| Dell Services Federal Government, Inc. | CDC Program Oversight & Implementation | GA | 375,000 |
| Deloitte Consulting, LLP | Project Management Contract Support | GA | 200,000 |
| Northrop Grumman | Community Transformation Grants – Program Management | GA | 200,000 |
| Deloitte Consulting, LLP | CDC Program Oversight & Implementation | GA | 103,286 |
| Various – Emory University, JP Morgan Chase, Northrop Grumman | Contracts < $25K | GA | 19,489 |
| DOE IAA | CDC Program Oversight & Implementation | GA | 12,000 |
| **Total** | | | **$31,364,071** |

Source: GAO analysis of HHS information.

**Activity**: Section 317 Immunization Program

The purpose of this activity is to provide funding for immunization operations and infrastructure necessary to implement a comprehensive immunization program at the federal, state, and local levels.

- **Fiscal year 2010**: None

- **Fiscal year 2011**: $99.8 million (73 grants in six funding announcements totaling $46.5 million and contracts totaling $53.3 million)

**Table 15: FY 2011 Grants, Section 317 Immunization Program**

| Announcements (6) | Recipient | State | Award (dollars) |
|---|---|---|---|
| 1. Competitive Program Expansion Supplement for CDC-RFA-HM08-805: Strengthen and Improve the Nation's Capacity through National, Non-profit, Professional Public Health Organizations to Increase Health Protection and Health Equity (CDC-RFA-HM08-8050402PHFF11) | National Association of City/County Health Officials | DC | $200,000 |
| | **Total (1 award)** | | **$200,000** |
| **Purpose (award type)**: To support the provision of capacity building assistance to state, tribal, local and territorial health departments that ensures performance improvement and successful adoption of best or promising practices to address key areas of public health infrastructure investments. (Supplement) | | | |
| **Legislative Authority**: Sections 301 and 317 of the Public Health Service Act (PHS Act), 42 USC, 241 and 247b as amended. Funding is appropriated under the Affordable Care Act (PL 111-148), Title IV, Section 4002 (Prevention and Public Health Fund). | | | |
| **Eligibility**: Limited to specific national, non-profit, public health professional organizations funded through the competitive funding opportunity announcement CDC-RFA-HM08-805. | | | |
| 2. Prevention and Public Health Fund: Capacity Building Assistance to Strengthen Public Health Immunization Infrastructure and Performance (CDC-RFA-IP11-1107PPHF11) | Arkansas State Dept of Health | AR | $3,586,942 |
| | Kansas State Dept of Hlth and Environmnt | KS | 3,115,885 |
| | New York State Dept of Health | NY | 2,573,336 |
| **Purpose (award type)**: To assist Section 317 grantees' transitions into a health care environment that is being transformed by the Affordable Care Act. (New) | Massachusetts State Dept of Pub Health | MA | 2,570,827 |
| | Colorado State Dept/Pub Hlth & Environmt | CO | 1,800,000 |
| | Washington State Department of Health | WA | 1,736,427 |
| **Legislative Authority**: Sections 301 and 317 of the Public Health Service Act (PHS Act), 42 USC, 241 and 247b as amended and the Patient Protection and Affordable Care Act (PL 111-148). | Connecticut State Dept of Public Health | CT | 1,611,744 |
| | Alabama State Dept of Public Health | AL | 1,438,016 |
| | Missouri State Dept/Health & Senior Srv | MO | 1,397,940 |
| **Eligibility**: Limited to grantees that are currently funded under funding announcement RFP IP08-803 because they have the necessary infrastructure in place to perform the activities required and have the experience needed to successfully complete the required functions. | West Virginia State Dept Hlth/Human Rscs | WV | 1,317,124 |
| | Maryland State Dept of Hlth/Mtl Hygiene | MD | 1,297,548 |
| | Minnesota State Dept of Health | MN | 1,261,172 |
| | Maine State Dept/Health/Human Servs | ME | 1,256,896 |
| | Michigan State Dept of Community Health | MI | 1,235,590 |
| | Arizona State Department of Hlth Srvcs | AZ | 1,162,818 |
| | Oklahoma State Department of Health | OK | 1,046,675 |
| | Georgia Department of Community Health | GA | 1,036,494 |
| | North Carolina State Dept/Hlth & Human Services | NC | 1,023,484 |

| Announcements (6) | Recipient | State | Award (dollars) |
|---|---|---|---|
| | Hawaii State Department of Health | HI | 933,189 |
| | Iowa State Dept of Public Health | IA | 900,000 |
| | New Jersey State Dept/Health/Senior Srvs | NJ | 876,197 |
| | Vermont Department of Health | VT | 792,138 |
| | California Department of Public Health | CA | 765,000 |
| | Wisconsin Department of Health Services | WI | 756,548 |
| | Florida State Department of Health | FL | 718,920 |
| | South Carolina State Dept of Hlth/Env | SC | 654,034 |
| | Oregon State Public Health Division | OR | 639,590 |
| | Texas State Dept of Health Services | TX | 540,000 |
| | Nevada State Dept of Hlth/Human Svcs | NV | 539,989 |
| | Utah State Department of Health | UT | 515,979 |
| | Nebraska St Dept of Health & Human Servs | NE | 492,300 |
| | Wyoming State Department of Health | WY | 485,906 |
| | Mississippi State Department of Health | MS | 484,195 |
| | Virginia State Dept of Health | VA | 452,061 |
| | Indiana State Department of Health | IN | 271,141 |
| | Ohio State Department of Health | OH | 252,275 |
| | North Dakota State Department of Health | ND | 226,418 |
| | Houston City Health & Human Services | TX | 134,842 |
| | **Total (38 awards)** | | **$41,899,640** |
| 3. Enhanced Surveillance for New Vaccine Preventable Disease (RFA-IP-11-010)<br><br>**Purpose (award type)**: To establish surveillance and evaluation sites that will collaborate as a larger network as the New vaccine Surveillance Network to conduct multi-site and individual projects to assess the impact of new vaccines and vaccine policies for diseases among children that are currently vaccine-preventable and those that are potentially vaccine preventable in the future. (New)<br><br>**Legislative Authority**: Sections 317(k)(1) of the Public Health Service Act as amended (42 U.S.C. 247b(k)(1)). | University of Rochester | NY | $201,220 |
| | The Children's Mercy Hospital | MO | 201,220 |
| | Cincinnati Children's Hospital | OH | 201,220 |
| | Vanderbilt University Medical Center | TN | 201,220 |
| | Seattle Children's Hospital | WA | 201,220 |
| | **Total (5 awards)** | | **$1,006,100** |

| Announcements (6) | Recipient | State | Award (dollars) |
|---|---|---|---|
| **Eligibility**: Eligible applicants include higher education institutions, nonprofits, independent school districts, housing authorities, faith-based, community-based, and regional organizations, Bona Fide agents, and state, county, city or township, special districts, federally and nonfederally recognized tribal, and U.S. territory or possession governments. Entities must be states (or bona fide agents to states), political subdivisions of states, or other public or non-profit private entities. | | | |
| 4. Patient Protection and Affordable Care Act (ACA), Emerging Infections Programs (EIP), Enhancing Epidemiology and Laboratory Capacity (CDC- RFA-CI10-00302PPHF11) | New York State Dept of Health | NY | $409,254 |
| | California Department of Public Health | CA | 381,103 |
| | Minnesota State Dept of Health | MN | 328,791 |
| **Purpose (award type)**: The purpose of the EIP-ACA cooperative agreement is to support state and local health departments' surveillance infrastructure through enhancement of the epidemiology and laboratory capacity of existing EIP network. (Continuation) | Georgia Department of Community Health | GA | 212,612 |
| | Connecticut State Dept of Public Health | CT | 199,515 |
| | Colorado State Dept/Pub Hlth & Environmt | CO | 191,878 |
| | Oregon State Public Health Division | OR | 167,139 |
| **Legislative Authority**: Sections 301(a) [42 U.S.C. 241(a)] and 317(k) (2) [42 U.S.C. 247b (k) (2)] of the Public Health Service Act, as amended and the Patient Protection and Affordable Care Act (PPACA) (Public Law 111-148), Title IV, Sections 4002 and 4304 (Prevention and Public Health Fund). | Tennessee State Department of Health | TN | 162,890 |
| | New Mexico State Department of Health | NM | 162,131 |
| | Maryland State Dept of Hlth/Mtl Hygiene | MD | 145,460 |
| | **Total (10 awards)** | | **$2,360,773** |
| **Eligibility**: Limited to health departments of states (or bona fide agents) currently funded under funding announcement CI10-003. | | | |
| 5. Patient Protection and Affordable Care Act (ACA), Emerging Infections Programs (EIP) (CI05-0026) | Georgia Department of Public Health | GA | $253,635 |
| | CT ST Dept of Public Health | CT | 154,877 |
| **Purpose (award type)**: To provide continued support to Emerging Infections Programs. (Continuation) | **Total (2 awards)** | | **$408,512** |
| **Legislative Authority**: Sections 301(a) [42 U.S.C. 241(a)], 317(k) (1) [42 U.S.C. 247b (k) (1)], and 317 (k) (2) [42 U.S.C. 247b (k) (2)], as amended. | | | |
| **Eligibility**: Limited to state governments or their bona fide agents. | | | |

| Announcements (6) | Recipient | State | Award (dollars) |
|---|---|---|---|
| 6. Patient Protection and Affordable Care Act Epidemiology and Laboratory Capacity for Infectious Diseases (ELC) Building and Strengthening Epidemiology, Laboratory and Health Information Systems Capacity in State and Local Health Departments (CDC-RFA-CI10–101202PPHF11)<br><br>**Purpose (award type)**: To enhance public health programs to improve health and help restrain the rate of growth of health care costs through building epidemiology, laboratory, and health information systems capacity in state and local public health departments. (Continuation)<br><br>**Legislative Authority**: Sections 301(a) [42 U.S.C. 241(a)] and 317(k) (2) [42 U.S.C. 247b (k) (2)] of the Public Health Service Act, as amended and the Patient Protection and Affordable Care Act (PL 111-148), Title IV, Sections 4002 and 4304 (Prevention and Public Health Fund).<br><br>**Eligibility**: Limited to 58 current Epidemiology and Laboratory Capacity for Infectious Disease Affordable Care Act state and local public health department grantees or their bona fide agents of funding announcement CI10-1012. | Los Angeles County Health Services Dept | CA | $124,611 |
|  | Utah State Department of Health | UT | 63,409 |
|  | New York City Health/Mental Hygiene | NY | 39,963 |
|  | Maine State Dept/Health/Human Servs | ME | 35,624 |
|  | Iowa State Dept of Public Health | IA | 35,000 |
|  | Washington State Department of Health | WA | 34,659 |
|  | Massachusetts State Dept of Pub Health | MA | 32,450 |
|  | Arizona State Department of Hlth Srvcs | AZ | 26,996 |
|  | NC State Dept/Hlth & Human Services | NC | 26,798 |
|  | South Carolina State Dept of Hlth/Env | SC | 26,624 |
|  | Florida State Department of Health | FL | 26,190 |
|  | Houston City Health & Human Services | TX | 26,000 |
|  | Wisconsin Department of Health Services | WI | 25,744 |
|  | Tennessee State Department of Health | TN | 23,943 |
|  | Alabama State Dept of Public Health | AL | 23,340 |
|  | Oklahoma State Department of Health | OK | 17,016 |
|  | City of Philadelphia Public Health Dept | PA | 17,000 |
|  | **Total (17awards)** |  | **$605,367** |

Source: GAO analysis of HHS information.

**Table 16: FY 2011 Contracts, Section 317 Immunization Program**

| Recipient | Purpose | State | Award (dollars) |
|---|---|---|---|
| Merck Sharp & Dohme Corp. | Vaccine Supplies | GA | $20,523,444 |
| Pfizer Inc. | Vaccine Supplies | GA | 6,817,823 |
| Sanofi Pasteur Inc. | Vaccine Supplies | GA | 5,751,222 |
| Glaxosmithkline LLC | Vaccine Supplies | GA | 4,843,178 |
| Merck Sharp & Dohme Corp. | Vaccine Supplies | GA | 4,413,348 |
| Deloitte Consulting, LLP | Barcoding - Implementation Pilot for Two-Dimensional Vaccine Barcode Utilization | GA | 2,907,887 |
| Glaxosmithkline LLC | Vaccine Supplies | GA | 2,858,200 |
| Four Seasons Environmental, Inc. | CDC Program Oversight & Implementation | GA | 2,149,345 |
| Novartis Vaccines and Diagnostics, Inc. | Vaccine Supplies | GA | 565,969 |
| Northrup Grumman Systems Corporation | IIS-TIPS | GA | 446,831 |
| The Cadence Group, Inc. | PPHF project management | GA | 415,758 |
| Carter Consulting, Inc. | VTrckS-IIS interface | GA | 410,363 |
| Carter Consulting, Inc. | Billing Planning and Implementation - Technical Assistance Management of NCIRD funded grants Support for the Education, Information, and Partnership Branch (EIPB), Immunization Services Division (ISD), National Center for Immunization and Respiratory Diseases (NCIRD) | GA | 340,952 |
| P3S Corporation | Evaluation of PCV 13 Vaccine - RBD Contractors | GA | 263,017 |
| Novartis Vaccines and Diagnostics, Inc. | Vaccine Supplies | GA | 190,861 |
| P3S Corporation | Enhanced Pertussis Surveillance and Eval of Acellular VE | GA | 164,044 |
| P3S Corporation | Strengthening the Evidence Base - MCV Evaluation - MVDB Contractors | GA | 81,820 |
| Agilent Technologies, Applied Biosystems Bio-Rad Laboratories, Caliper Life Sciences, J P Morgan Chase Bank, Roche Diagnostics Corporation | Contracts < $25K | N/A | 73,165 |
| GSA Federal Telecommunication Service | Evaluation Impact and Effectiveness of Rotavirus Vaccine | GA | 50,200 |
| MA Biological Laboratory | Vaccine Supplies | GA | 35,955 |
| Southeast Scientific | Maintenance of 35 freezers | GA | 33,557 |
| Goodwill Industries of North GA | CDC Program Oversight & Implementation | GA | 10,655 |
| **Total** | | | **$53,347,594** |

Source: GAO analysis of HHS information.

**Activity**: National Public Health Improvement Initiative

The purpose of this activity[2] is to systematically increase the capacity of public health departments to detect and respond to public health events requiring highly coordinated interventions to improve and/or sustain the performance (efficiency/effectiveness) of public health organizations, systems, practices, and essential services. It is intended to promote the development, dissemination, and adoption of evidence-based practices.

- **Fiscal year 2010**: $47.9 million (80 grants in two funding announcements totaling $46.4 million and three contracts totaling $1.5 million)

- **Fiscal year 2011**: $40.2 million (80 grants in three funding announcements totaling $36.7 million and four contracts totaling $3.5 million)

---

[2]According to HHS, this activity was called Public Health Infrastructure in fiscal year 2010.

Table 17: FY 2010 Grants, National Public Health Improvement Initiative

| Announcements (2) | Recipient | State | Award (dollars) |
|---|---|---|---|
| 1. Strengthening Public Health Infrastructure for Improved Health Outcomes (CDC-RFA-CD10-1011) | California Department of Public Health | CA | $2,060,128 |
| | Florida State Department of Health | FL | 2,060,128 |
| **Purpose (award type)**: To support innovative changes in key areas that improve the quality, effectiveness and efficiency of the public health infrastructure that will support the delivery of public health services and programs as specified within the Affordable Care Act. (New) | New York City Health/Mental Hygiene | NY | 2,060,128 |
| | Wisconsin Department of Health Services | WI | 1,960,129 |
| | Massachusetts State Dept of Pub Health | MA | 1,960,128 |
| | Minnesota State Dept of Health | MN | 1,960,128 |
| **Legislative Authority**: Sections 301 and 317 of the Public Health Service Act (PHS Act), 42 USC, 241 and 247b as amended. Funding is appropriated under the Affordable Care Act (PL 111-148), Title IV, Section 4002 (Prevention and Public Health Fund). | North Carolina State Dept/Hlth & Human Services | NC | 1,903,858 |
| | Oregon State Public Health Division | OR | 1,860,128 |
| | Los Angeles County Health Services Dept | CA | 1,859,950 |
| | Cherokee Nation | OK | 1,760,128 |
| **Eligibility**: All 50 states, Washington D.C., 9 large local health departments supporting cities with populations of 1 million or more inhabitants, 5 U.S. Territories, 3 U.S. Affiliated Pacific Islands and up to 7 federally recognized tribes (or their equivalent) with an established public health department structure that provide public health services. | Maine State Dept/Health/Human Servs | ME | 1,758,786 |
| | Pacific Islands Health Officers Assn | HI | 1,660,128 |
| | New Jersey State Dept/Health/Senior Srvs | NJ | 1,638,751 |
| | Tennessee State Department of Health | TN | 1,296,995 |
| | Nebraska St Dept of Health & Human Servs | NE | 1,200,000 |
| | West Virginia State Dept Hlth/Human Rscs | WV | 1,200,000 |
| | City of Philadelphia Public Health Dept | PA | 1,118,493 |
| | Hawaii State Department of Health | HI | 1,100,000 |
| | Vermont Department of Health | VT | 1,100,000 |
| | Illinois State Dept of Public Health | IL | 400,000 |
| | Michigan State Dept of Community Health | MI | 400,000 |
| | New York State Dept of Health | NY | 400,000 |
| | Pennsylvania State Dept of Health | PA | 400,000 |
| | Texas State Dept of Health Services | TX | 400,000 |
| | Georgia Department of Community Health | GA | 399,836 |
| | Ohio State Department of Health | OH | 394,111 |
| | Colorado State Dept/Pub Hlth & Environmt | CO | 300,000 |
| | Indiana State Department of Health | IN | 300,000 |
| | Maryland State Dept of Hlth/Mtl Hygiene | MD | 300,000 |
| | Missouri State Dept/Health & Senior Srv | MO | 300,000 |
| | Virginia State Dept of Health | VA | 300,000 |
| | Washington State Department of Health | WA | 299,981 |
| | Arizona State Department of Hlth Srvcs | AZ | 289,586 |
| | Alabama State Dept of Public Health | AL | 200,000 |
| | Arkansas State Dept of Health | AR | 200,000 |

| Announcements (2) | Recipient | State | Award (dollars) |
|---|---|---|---|
| | Connecticut State Dept of Public Health | CT | 200,000 |
| | Idaho State Dept of Health and Welfare | ID | 200,000 |
| | City of Chicago | IL | 200,000 |
| | Iowa State Dept of Public Health | IA | 200,000 |
| | Kansas State Dept of Hlth and Environmnt | KS | 200,000 |
| | KY Cabinet for Health and Family Services | KY | 200,000 |
| | Louisiana State Dept of Hlth & Hospitals | LA | 200,000 |
| | Nevada State Dept of Hlth/Human Svcs | NV | 200,000 |
| | Oklahoma State Department of Health | OK | 200,000 |
| | Puerto Rico Department of Health | PR | 200,000 |
| | South Carolina State Dept of Hlth/Env | SC | 200,000 |
| | Houston City Health & Human Services | TX | 200,000 |
| | Utah State Department of Health | UT | 200,000 |
| | New Mexico State Department of Health | NM | 199,877 |
| | Mississippi State Department of Health | MS | 199,585 |
| | County of Maricopa | AZ | 199,434 |
| | Alaska State Department of Hlth-Soc Svcs | AK | 100,000 |
| | Alaska Native Tribal Health Consortium | AK | 100,000 |
| | Southeast Alaska Reg Hlth Consortium | AK | 100,000 |
| | American Samoa Department of Health | AS | 100,000 |
| | Gila River Indian Community | AZ | 100,000 |
| | Navajo Nation Division of Health | AZ | 100,000 |
| | County/San Diego Health / Human Ser/Ag | CA | 100,000 |
| | DC Department of Health | DC | 100,000 |
| | Delaware State Dept of Hlth & Soc Srvs | DE | 100,000 |
| | Federated States Micronesia | FM | 100,000 |
| | Guam Department of Public Health-Soc Svc | GU | 100,000 |
| | Republic/Marshall Island Mnstry of Hlth | MH | 100,000 |
| | Montana State Dept/Pub Hlth & Human Srvs | MT | 100,000 |
| | Montana-Wyoming Tribal Leaders Council | MT | 100,000 |
| | Commonwealth N Mariana Is Dept Pub Hlth | MP | 100,000 |
| | NH State Dept of Health and Human Sers | NH | 100,000 |
| | Northwest Portland Area Indian Hlth Bd | OR | 100,000 |
| | City of San Antonio Metro Health Dist | TX | 100,000 |
| | Dallas County Dept/Hlth/Human Srvs | TX | 100,000 |
| | Virgin Islands Department of Health | VI | 100,000 |

| Announcements (2) | Recipient | State | Award (dollars) |
|---|---|---|---|
| | Wyoming State Department of Health | WY | 100,000 |
| | Republic/Marshall Island Mnstry of Hlth | MH | 100,000 |
| | Mille Lacs Band of Ojibwe Indians | MN | 99,866 |
| | Rhode Island State Dept of Health | RI | 99,738 |
| | **Total (75 awards)** | | **$42,400,000** |
| 2. Competitive Supplement to CDC-RFA-HM08-805: Strengthen and Improve the Nation's Capacity through National, Non-profit, Professional Public Health Organizations to Increase Health Protection and Health Equity (CDC-RFA-HM08-8050301SUPP10) | National Network of Public Health Institutes | LA | $1,000,000 |
| | American Public Health Association | DC | 750,000 |
| | National Association of City/County Health Officials | DC | 750,000 |
| | Public Health Foundation | DC | 750,000 |
| | Association of State and Territorial Health Officials | VA | 750,000 |
| **Purpose (award type)**: To support the provision of capacity building assistance to state, tribal, local and territorial health departments that ensures successful adoption of best or promising practices to address key areas of public health infrastructure investments. (Supplement) | **Total (5 awards)** | | **$4,000,000** |

**Purpose (award type)**: To support the provision of capacity building assistance to state, tribal, local and territorial health departments that ensures successful adoption of best or promising practices to address key areas of public health infrastructure investments. (Supplement)

**Legislative Authority**: Sections 301 and 317 of the Public Health Service Act (PHS Act), 42 USC, 241 and 247b as amended. Funding is appropriated under the Affordable Care Act (PL 111-148), Title IV, Section 4002 (Prevention and Public Health Fund).

**Eligibility**: Limited to specific national, non-profit, public health professional organizations funded through the funding announcement CDC-RFA-HM08-805.

Source: GAO analysis of HHS information.

Note: In fiscal year 2010, this activity was referred to as Public Health Infrastructure.

**Table 18: FY 2010 Contracts, National Public Health Improvement Initiative**

| Recipient | Purpose | State | Award (dollars) |
|---|---|---|---|
| Office of Personnal Management | Competencies necessary for Workforce | GA | $1,500,000 |
| Deloitte Consulting, LLP | Business services support - Health Reform Implementation Office | GA | 12,358 |
| Northrop Grumman | Support all aspects of full lifecycle application systems development and maintenance on a variety of platforms including mainframe, client server, and web; architecture and infrastructure design to support enterprise application software services including hardware/software/network design and implementation; database design, application development and support; data management and security controls; quality assurance, test and control functions; and technical communication, consultation and information support. | GA | 7,000 |
| Total (3 awards) | | | $1,519,358 |

Source: GAO analysis of HHS information.

Note: In fiscal year 2010, this activity was referred to as Public Health Infrastructure.

**Table 19: FY 2011 Grants, National Public Health Improvement Initiative**

| Announcements (3) | Recipient | State | Award (dollars) |
|---|---|---|---|
| 1. Public Prevention Health Fund: Strengthening Public Health Infrastructure for Improved Health Outcomes (CDC-RFA-CD10-101101PPHF11)<br><br>**Purpose (award type)**: To provide support for accelerating public health accreditation readiness activities; to provide additional support for performance management and improvement practices; and, for the development, identification and dissemination of evidence-based policies and practices. (Supplement)<br><br>**Legislative Authority**: Sections 301 and 317 of the Public Health Service Act (PHS Act), 42 USC, 241 and 247b as amended. Funding is appropriated under the Affordable Care Act (PL 111-148), Title IV, Section 4002 (Prevention and Public Health Fund).<br><br>**Eligibility**: Limited to 76 official public health agencies that are current recipients of project grants for Strengthening Public Health Infrastructure for Improved Health Outcomes under funding opportunity CDC-RFA-CD10-1011. | New York City Health/Mental Hygiene | NY | $1,093,662 |
| | Florida State Department of Health | FL | 1,093,662 |
| | California Department of Public Health | CA | 1,093,662 |
| | NC State Dept/Hlth & Human Services | NC | 1,037,779 |
| | Minnesota State Dept of Health | MN | 993,662 |
| | Wisconsin Department of Health Services | WI | 993,662 |
| | Massachusetts State Dept of Pub Health | MA | 993,662 |
| | New Jersey State Dept/Health/Senior Srvs | NJ | 950,791 |
| | Oregon State Public Health Division | OR | 893,662 |
| | Los Angeles County Health Services Dept | CA | 893,598 |
| | Cherokee Nation | OK | 843,662 |
| | Maine State Dept/Health/Human Servs | ME | 843,182 |
| | Tennessee State Department of Health | TN | 757,600 |
| | City of Philadelphia Public Health Dept | PA | 664,213 |
| | Nebraska St Dept of Health & Human Servs | NE | 657,600 |
| | West Virginia State Dept Hlth/Human Rscs | WV | 657,600 |
| | Hawaii State Department of Health | HI | 607,600 |
| | Vermont Department of Health | VT | 607,600 |
| | Pacific Islands Health Officers Assn | HI | 593,662 |
| | Pennsylvania State Dept of Health | PA | 500,000 |
| | New York State Dept of Health | NY | 500,000 |
| | Illinois State Dept of Public Health | IL | 500,000 |
| | Michigan State Dept of Community Health | MI | 500,000 |
| | Ohio State Department of Health | OH | 500,000 |
| | Texas State Dept of Health Services | TX | 500,000 |
| | Georgia Department of Community Health | GA | 499,738 |
| | Maryland State Dept of Hlth/Mtl Hygiene | MD | 400,000 |
| | Missouri State Dept/ Health & Senior Srv | MO | 400,000 |
| | Indiana State Department of Health | IN | 400,000 |
| | Washington State Department of Health | WA | 400,000 |
| | Colorado State Dept/Pub Hlth & Environmt | CO | 400,000 |
| | Arizona State Department of Hlth Srvcs | AZ | 400,000 |
| | Virgnia State Dept of Health | VA | 399,859 |
| | Arkansas State Dept of Health | AR | 300,000 |
| | City of Chicago | IL | 300,000 |

| Announcements (3) | Recipient | State | Award (dollars) |
| --- | --- | --- | --- |
| | Houston City Health & Human Services | TX | 300,000 |
| | Alabama State Dept of Public Health | AL | 300,000 |
| | County of Maricopa | AZ | 300,000 |
| | Kansas State Dept of Hlth and Environmnt | KS | 300,000 |
| | KY Cabinet for Health and Family Services | KY | 300,000 |
| | Louisiana State Dept of Hlth & Hospitals | LA | 300,000 |
| | Nevada State Dept of Hlth/Human Svcs | NV | 300,000 |
| | Idaho State Dept of Health and Welfare | ID | 300,000 |
| | Oklahoma State Department of Health | OK | 300,000 |
| | Utah State Department of Health | UT | 300,000 |
| | Connecticut State Dept of Public Health | CT | 300,000 |
| | Iowa State Dept of Public Health | IA | 300,000 |
| | New Mexico State Department of Health | NM | 300,000 |
| | Puerto Rico Department of Health | PR | 300,000 |
| | South Carolina State Dept of Hlth/Env | SC | 300,000 |
| | Mississippi State Department of Health | MS | 299,585 |
| | County/San Diego Health / Human Ser/Ag | CA | 250,000 |
| | DC Department of Health | DC | 250,000 |
| | Delaware State Dept of Hlth & Soc Srvs | DE | 250,000 |
| | NH State Dept of Health and Human Sers | NH | 250,000 |
| | Northwest Portland Area Indian Hlth Bd | OR | 250,000 |
| | City of San Antonio Metro Health Dist | TX | 250,000 |
| | Alaska State Department of Hlth-Soc Svcs | AK | 250,000 |
| | Rhode Island State Dept of Health | RI | 250,000 |
| | Navajo Nation Division of Health | AZ | 250,000 |
| | Alaska Native Tribal Health Consortium | AK | 250,000 |
| | American Samoa Department of Health | AS | 250,000 |
| | Federated States Micronesia | FM | 250,000 |
| | Guam Department of Public Health-Soc Svc | GU | 250,000 |
| | Mille Lacs Band of Ojibwe Indians | MN | 250,000 |
| | Republic/Marshall Island Mnstry of Hlth | MH | 250,000 |
| | Montana WY Tribal Leaders Council | MT | 250,000 |
| | MT State Dept/Pub Hlth & Human Srvs | MT | 250,000 |
| | Republic of Palau Ministry of Health | PW | 250,000 |
| | Southeast Alaska Reg Hlth Consortium | AK | 250,000 |
| | Dallas County Dept/Hlth/Human Srvs | TX | 249,998 |
| | Commonwealth N Mariana Is Dept Pub Hlth | MP | 249,993 |

| Announcements (3) | Recipient | State | Award (dollars) |
|---|---|---|---|
| | Wyoming State Department of Health | WY | 248,838 |
| | Gila River Indian Community | AZ | 100,000 |
| | **Total (74 awards)** | | **$33,568,532** |
| 2. Competitive Program Expansion Supplement for CDC-RFA-HM08-805: Strengthen and Improve the Nation's Capacity through National, Non-profit, Professional Public Health Organizations to Increase Health Protection and Health Equity (CDC-RFA-HM08-8050402PHFF11) | National Association of City/County Health Officials | DC | $300,000 |
| | **Total (1 award)** | | **$300,000** |
| **Purpose (award type)**: To support the provision of capacity building assistance to state, tribal, local and territorial health departments that ensures performance improvement and successful adoption of best or promising practices to address key areas of public health infrastructure investments. (Supplement) | | | |
| **Legislative Authority**: Sections 301 and 317 of the Public Health Service Act (PHS Act), 42 USC, 241 and 247b as amended. Funding is appropriated under the Affordable Care Act (PL 111-148), Title IV, Section 4002 (Prevention and Public Health Fund). | | | |
| **Eligibility**: Limited to specific national, non-profit, public health professional organizations funded through the competitive funding opportunity announcement CDC-RFA-HM08-805. | | | |
| 3. Non-Competitive 12-month Cost Extension Supplement for CDC-RFA-HM08-8050301SUPP10: Affordable Care Act (ACA): Capacity Building Assistance to Strengthen Public Health Infrastructure and Performance (CDC-RFA-HM08-8050401PPHF11) | National Association of City/County Health Officials | DC | $999,400 |
| | American Public Health Association | DC | 464,400 |
| | Public Health Foundation | DC | 464,400 |
| | National Network of Public Health Institutes | LA | 464,400 |
| | Association of State and Territorial Health Officials | VA | 464,400 |
| **Purpose (award type)**: To support the provision of capacity building assistance to state, tribal, local and territorial health departments that ensures performance improvement and successful adoption of best or promising practices to address key areas of public health infrastructure investments. (Supplement) | **Total (5 awards)** | | **$2,857,000** |
| **Legislative Authority**: Sections 301 and 317 of the Public Health Service Act (PHS Act), 42 USC, 241 and 247b as amended. Funding is appropriated under the Affordable Care Act (PL 111-148), Title IV, Section 4002 (Prevention and Public Health Fund). | | | |
| **Eligibility**: Limited to specific national, non-profit, public health professional organizations funded under CDC-RFA-HM08-8030301SUPP10 funding opportunity announcement. | | | |

Source: GAO analysis of HHS information.

**Table 20: FY 2011 Contracts, National Public Health Improvement Initiative**

| Recipient | Purpose | State | Award (dollars) |
|---|---|---|---|
| Deloitte Consulting, LLP | National Public Health Improvement Initiative (NPHII) Implementation Support | GA | $1,751,979 |
| Goodwill Industries of North Georgia | CDC Program Oversight & Implementation | GA | 1,407,000 |
| Deloitte Consulting, LLP | CDC Program Oversight & Implementation | GA | 201,000 |
| Total Solutions, Inc. | Administrative Support | GA | 114,489 |
| **Total (4 awards)** | | | **$3,474,468** |

Source: GAO analysis of HHS information.

## Activity: Tobacco Prevention (Media and Quitlines)

The purpose of this activity is to raise awareness and shift key attitudes and beliefs about the harms of tobacco use and exposure to secondhand smoke in areas of the country with some of the highest rates of tobacco use prevalence.

- **Fiscal year 2010**: $14.1 million (46 grants in two funding announcements totaling $3.9 million and seven contracts totaling $10.2 million)

- **Fiscal year 2011**: $49.1 million (43 grants in two funding announcements totaling $5.0 million and 11 contracts totaling $44.1million)

## Table 21: FY 2010 Grants, Tobacco Prevention (Media and Quitlines)

| Announcements (2) | Recipient | State | Award (dollars) |
|---|---|---|---|
| 1. Patient Protection and Affordable Care Act: State Supplemental Funding for Healthy Communities, Tobacco Prevention and Control, Diabetes Prevention and Control, and Behavioral Risk Factor Surveillance System (RFA-DP09-90101SUPP10)<br><br>**Purpose (award type)**: To provide additional financial and programmatic assistance to strengthen the abilities of States, the District of Columbia, and eligible U.S. Territories to move towards implementing a plan to reduce tobacco use through legislative, regulatory, and educational arenas, as well as enhance and expand the national network of tobacco cessation quitlines to significantly increase the number of tobacco users who quit each year to reduce mortality and morbidity from tobacco use, and associated health care costs. (Supplement)<br><br>**Legislative Authority**: Sections 301, 307, 310, and 311 of the Public Health Service Act, as amended, and the Comprehensive Smoking Education Act of 1984, Comprehensive Smokeless Tobacco Health Education Act of 1986, and the American Recovery and Reinvestment Act of 2009 (Recovery Act) [Public Law 111-5].<br><br>**Eligibility**: Eligibility is limited to state agencies, the District of Columbia, and U.S. Territories that are funded under funding announcement DP09-901. | California Department of Public Health | CA | $240,173 |
| | NC State Dept/Hlth & Human Services | NC | 198,758 |
| | New York State Dept of Health | NY | 150,543 |
| | Florida State Department of Health | FL | 145,380 |
| | Illinois State Dept of Public Health | IL | 116,426 |
| | Pennsylvania State Dept of Health | PA | 114,853 |
| | Ohio State Department of Health | OH | 109,388 |
| | Texas State Dept of Health Services | TX | 102,360 |
| | Michigan State Dept of Community Health | MI | 101,296 |
| | Georgia Department of Community Health | GA | 100,573 |
| | New Jersey State Dept/Health/Senior Srvs | NJ | 94,802 |
| | Virginia State Dept of Health | VA | 90,557 |
| | Washington State Department of Health | WA | 84,288 |
| | Arizona State Department of Hlth Srvcs | AZ | 83,936 |
| | Massachusetts State Dept of Pub Health | MA | 83,924 |
| | Indiana State Department of Health | IN | 83,048 |
| | Tennessee State Department of Health | TN | 82,395 |
| | Missouri State Dept/ Health & Senior Srv | MO | 80,807 |
| | Maryland State Dept of Hlth/Mtl Hygiene | MD | 79,325 |
| | Wisconsin Department of Health Services | WI | 79,095 |
| | Minnesota State Dept of Health | MN | 77,095 |
| | Alabama State Dept of Public Health | AL | 74,227 |
| | Colorado State Dept/Pub Hlth & Environmt | CO | 73,927 |
| | South Carolina State Dept of Hlth/Env | SC | 73,468 |
| | Louisiana State Dept of Hlth & Hospitals | LA | 73,112 |
| | KY Cabinet for Health and Family Services | KY | 72,033 |
| | Puerto Rico Department of Health | PR | 70,412 |
| | Oregon State Public Health Division | OR | 69,683 |
| | Oklahoma State Department of Health | OK | 68,970 |
| | Connecticut State Dept of Public Health | CT | 68,102 |
| | Iowa State Dept of Public Health | IA | 65,476 |
| | Arkansas State Dept of Health | AR | 64,867 |
| | Kansas State Dept of Hlth And Environmnt | KS | 64,045 |
| | Utah State Department of Health | UT | 63,874 |
| | Nevada State Dept of Hlth/Human Svcs | NV | 63,169 |

| Announcements (2) | Recipient | State | Award (dollars) |
|---|---|---|---|
| | New Mexico State Department of Health | NM | 60,340 |
| | West Virginia State Dept Hlth/Human Rscs | WV | 59,363 |
| | Nebraska St Dept of Health & Human Servs | NE | 59,244 |
| | Idaho State Dept of Health And Welfare | ID | 57,953 |
| | NH State Dept of Health And Human Sers | NH | 56,815 |
| | Delaware State Dept of Hlth & Soc Srvs | DE | 54,445 |
| | South Dakota State Dept of Health | SD | 54,180 |
| | Maine State Dept/Health/Human Servs | ME | 53,098 |
| | DC Department of Health | DC | 53,080 |
| | Wyoming State Department of Health | WY | 52,800 |
| | **Total (45 awards)** | | **$3,825,705** |
| 2. Patient Protection and Affordable Health Care Act (Affordable Care Act): Pacific Islands Supplemental Funding for Five-Year US Affiliated Pacific Island Collaborative Performance Agreement for Tobacco Control, Diabetes Prevention and Control, and the Behavioral Risk Factor Surveillance System (RFA-DP09-90201SUPP10). | Guam Department of Public Health-Soc Svc | GU | $50,000 |
| | **Total (1 award)** | | **$50,000** |

**Purpose (award type)**: To strengthen Guam's ability to move towards implementing a comprehensive plan to reduce tobacco use through legislative, regulatory, and educational arenas, as well to contribute to the enhancement and expansion of the national network of tobacco cessation quitlines to significantly increase the number of tobacco users who quit each year in order to reduce mortality and morbidity from tobacco use, and associated health care costs. (Supplement)

**Legislative Authority**: Section 301 (a), and 317 (k) (2) of the Public Health Service Act, [42 U.S.C. section 241 (a) and 247b (k) (2), as amended], and the Comprehensive Smoking Education Act of 1984, Comprehensive Smokeless Tobacco Health Education Act of 1986, and the American Recovery and Reinvestment Act of 2009 (Recovery Act) [Public Law 111-5].

**Eligibility**: Limited to Guam, which was funded under funding announcement DP09-902.

Source: GAO analysis of HHS information.

**Table 22: FY 2010 Contracts, Tobacco Prevention (Media and Quitlines)**

| Recipient | Purpose | State | Award (dollars) |
|---|---|---|---|
| Plowshare Group | Develop and implement a comprehensive communication and marketing plan to deliver actionable tobacco prevention information, messages, and interventions to the identified audience segments. | GA | $8,080,000 |
| MACRO | To provide health communications and integrated marketing strategies and database support to the Health Communications Branch, Office on Smoking and Health, NCCDPHP. | GA | 1,050,000 |
| Department of Health and Human Services | Plan, coordinate and deliver training and technical assistance to state and community health department staff and partners to support the implementation of policies leading to tobacco prevention and cessation. | MO | 539,344 |
| Plowshare Group | Develop and implement a comprehensive communication and marketing plan to deliver actionable tobacco prevention information, messages, and interventions to the identified audience segments. | GA | 347,044 |
| Deloitte Consulting, LLP | Business services support - Financial Management Office | GA | 180,000 |
| Deloitte Consulting, LLP | Business services support - Health Reform Implementation Office | GA | 30,000 |
| Deloitte Consulting, LLP | Business services support - Health Reform Implementation Office | GA | 20,000 |
| **Total (7 awards)** | | | **$10,246,388** |

Source: GAO analysis of HHS information.

**Table 23: FY 2011 Grants, Tobacco Prevention (Media and Quitlines)**

| Announcements (2) | Recipient | State | Award (dollars) |
|---|---|---|---|
| 1. State Supplemental Funding for Healthy Communities, Tobacco Prevention and Control, Diabetes Prevention and Control (CDC-RFA-DP09-9010201PPHF11)<br><br>**Purpose**: To provide additional financial and programmatic assistance to strengthen the abilities of states, the District of Columbia, and eligible U.S. Territories that were funded under Funding Announcement DP09-901 to reduce tobacco use through legislative, regulatory, and educational arenas, as well as enhance and expand the national network of tobacco cessation quitlines to significantly increase the number of tobacco users who quit each year to reduce mortality and morbidity from tobacco use, and associated health care costs. (Supplement)<br><br>**Legislative Authority**: Sections 301, 307, 310, and 311 of the Public Health Service Act, as amended, and the Comprehensive Smoking Education Act of 1984, Comprehensive Smokeless Tobacco Health Education Act of 1986, and the American Recovery and Reinvestment Act of 2009 (Recovery Act) [Public Law 111-5].<br><br>**Eligibility**: Eligibility is limited to State agencies, including the District of Columbia and U.S. Territories funded under announcement (DP09-901). | California Department of Public Health | CA | $340,245 |
| | Texas State Dept of Health Services | TX | 251,470 |
| | New York City Health/Mental Hygiene | NY | 213,269 |
| | Florida State Department of Health | FL | 205,000 |
| | Pennsylvania State Dept of Health | PA | 162,708 |
| | Ohio State Department of Health | OH | 154,966 |
| | Michigan State Dept of Community Health | MI | 143,503 |
| | NC State Dept/Hlth & Human Services | NC | 139,210 |
| | Virginia State Dept of Health | VA | 128,289 |
| | Washington State Department of Health | WA | 119,408 |
| | Arizona State Department of Hlth Srvcs | AZ | 118,909 |
| | Massachusetts State Dept of Pub Health | MA | 118,894 |
| | Indiana State Department of Health | IN | 117,651 |
| | Tennessee State Department of Health | TN | 116,726 |
| | Missouri State Dept/ Health & Senior Srv | MO | 114,477 |
| | Maryland State Dept of Hlth/Mtl Hygiene | MD | 112,377 |
| | Wisconsin Department of Health Services | WI | 112,051 |
| | Minnesota State Dept of Health | MN | 109,218 |
| | Colorado State Dept/Pub Hlth & Environmt | CO | 107,458 |
| | Alabama State Dept of Public Health | AL | 105,155 |
| | Louisiana State Dept of Hlth & Hospitals | LA | 103,575 |
| | KY Cabinet for Health and Family Services | KY | 102,279 |
| | Puerto Rico Department of Health | PR | 99,750 |
| | Oregon State Public Health Division | OR | 98,711 |
| | Oklahoma State Department of Health | OK | 97,707 |
| | Connecticut State Dept of Public Health | CT | 96,478 |
| | Iowa State Dept of Public Health | IA | 92,758 |
| | Arkansas State Dept of Health | AR | 91,895 |
| | Kansas State Dept of Hlth and Environmnt | KS | 91,379 |
| | Utah State Department of Health | UT | 91,130 |
| | Nevada State Dept of Hlth/Human Svcs | NV | 90,099 |
| | New Jersey State Dept/Health/Senior Srvs | NJ | 85,482 |
| | West Virginia State Dept Hlth/Human Rscs | WV | 84,098 |
| | Idaho State Dept of Health and Welfare | ID | 82,100 |
| | NH State Dept of Health and Human Sers | NH | 80,488 |

| Announcements (2) | Recipient | State | Award (dollars) |
|---|---|---|---|
| | Maine State Dept/Health/Human Servs | ME | 80,443 |
| | Hawaii State Department of Health | HI | 80,274 |
| | Rhode Island State Dept of Health | RI | 78,510 |
| | Montana State Dept/Pub Hlth & Human Srvs | MT | 77,939 |
| | Delaware State Dept of Hlth & Soc Srvs | DE | 77,285 |
| | Vermont Department of Health | VT | 75,365 |
| | Wyoming State Department of Health | WY | 74,800 |
| | **Total (42 awards)** | | **$4,923,529** |
| 2. Pacific Islands Supplemental Funding for Five-Year US Affiliated Pacific Island Collaborative Performance Agreement for Tobacco Control, Diabetes Prevention and Control (CDC-RFA-DP09-9020302PPHF11) | Guam Department of Public Health-Soc Svc | GU | $50,000 |
| | **Total (1 award)** | | **$50,000** |

**Purpose (award type)**: To create additional tobacco quitters, beyond what Guam has projected to achieve in Recovery Act funded programs. (Supplement)

**Legislative Authority**: Sections 301, 307, 310, and 311 of the Public Health Service Act, as amended, and the Comprehensive Smoking Education Act of 1984, Comprehensive Smokeless Tobacco Health Education Act of 1986, and the American Recovery and Reinvestment Act of 2009 (Recovery Act) [Public Law 111-5].

**Eligibility**: Limited to Guam health department.

Source: GAO analysis of HHS information.

**Table 24: FY 2011 Contracts, Tobacco Prevention (Media and Quitlines)**

| Recipient | Purpose | State | Award (dollars) |
|---|---|---|---|
| Plowshare Group, Inc. | CDC's National Tobacco Prevention and Control Public Education Campaign | GA | $34,313,221 |
| Plowshare Group, Inc | CDC's National Tobacco Prevention and Control Public Education Campaign | GA | 3,330,978 |
| Research Triangle Institute | Evaluation of the National Tobacco Prevention and Control Public Education Campaign | GA | 2,935,310 |
| Four Seasons Environmental, Inc. | CDC Program Oversight & Implementation | GA | 816,000 |
| Macro International Inc. | Communication, Marketing, and Database Strategies, Services and Support to the Office on Smoking and Health, Health Communications Branch | GA | 702,448 |
| Northrop Grumman | CDC Program Oversight & Implementation | GA | 584,000 |
| HHS Program Support Center | CASU Tobacco Prevention Activities | GA | 527,053 |
| Deloitte Consulting, LLP | CDC Program Oversight & Implementation | GA | 344,355 |
| North American Quitline Consortium | North American Quitline | GA | 263,000 |
| Deloitte Consulting, LLP | CDC Program Oversight & Implementation | GA | 250,000 |
| Emory University | TTAC – Competency Development Task 9 | GA | 37,962 |
| **Total (11 awards)** | | | **$44,104,327** |

Source: GAO analysis of HHS information.

## Activity: Epidemiology and Laboratory Capacity Grants

The purpose of this activity is to enhance the ability of state, local, and territorial Epidemiology and Laboratory Capacity (ELC) and EIP grantees to strengthen and integrate capacity for detecting and responding to infectious diseases and other public health threats.

- **Fiscal year 2010**: $19.2 million (68 grants in two funding announcements)

- **Fiscal year 2011**: $40.0 million (68 grants in two funding announcements totaling $38.4 million and two contracts totaling $1.6 million)

**Table 25: FY 2010 Grants, Epidemiology and Laboratory Capacity Grants**

| Announcements (2) | Recipient | State | Award (dollars) |
|---|---|---|---|
| 1. Patient Protection and Affordable Care Act, Epidemiology and Laboratory Capacity for Infectious Diseases, Building and Strengthening Epidemiology, Laboratory and Health Information Systems Capacity in State and Local Health Departments (CDC-RFA-CI10-1012)<br><br>**Purpose (award type)**: To assist state public health agencies improve surveillance for, and response to, infectious diseases and other public health threats by (1) strengthening epidemiologic capacity; (2) enhancing laboratory practice; (3) improving information systems; and (4) developing and implementing prevention and control strategies. (New)<br><br>**Legislative Authority**: Sections 301(a) [42 U.S.C. 241(a)] and 317(k) (2) [42 U.S.C. 247b (k) (2)] of the Public Health Service Act, as amended and the Patient Protection and Affordable Care Act (PL 111-148), Title IV, Sections 4002 and 4304 (Prevention and Public Health Fund).<br><br>**Eligibility**: Limited to 58 state and local public health agencies grantees who received funding through the Epidemiology and Laboratory Capacity for Infectious Diseases funding announcement CI04-040. | California Department of Public Health | CA | $677,043 |
| | Massachusetts State Dept of Pub Health | MA | 598,230 |
| | Illinois State Dept of Public Health | IL | 586,815 |
| | Texas State Dept of Health Services | TX | 544,902 |
| | Washington State Department of Health | WA | 510,120 |
| | Indiana State Department of Health | IN | 493,938 |
| | Arkansas State Dept of Health | AR | 442,594 |
| | Florida State Department of Health | FL | 423,403 |
| | Alaska State Department of Hlth-Soc Svcs | AK | 413,558 |
| | Los Angeles County Health Services Dept | CA | 412,980 |
| | Iowa State Dept of Public Health | IA | 407,337 |
| | Wisconsin Department of Health Services | WI | 395,014 |
| | KY Cabinet for Health and Family Services | KY | 389,385 |
| | New York State Dept of Health | NY | 374,166 |
| | Alabama State Dept of Public Health | AL | 361,795 |
| | Utah State Department of Health | UT | 352,662 |
| | New Jersey State Dept/Health/Senior Srvs | NJ | 346,382 |
| | New York City Health/Mental Hygiene | NY | 340,392 |
| | Colorado State Dept/Pub Hlth & Environmt | CO | 327,908 |
| | New Mexico State Department of Health | NM | 326,168 |
| | Montana State Dept/Pub Hlth & Human Srvs | MT | 312,811 |
| | Tennessee State Department of Health | TN | 308,225 |
| | Delaware State Dept of Hlth & Soc Srvs | DE | 307,243 |
| | Minnesota State Dept of Health | MN | 304,209 |
| | MS State Department of Health | MS | 302,720 |
| | Ohio State Department of Health | OH | 298,394 |
| | Rhode Island State Dept of Health | RI | 296,803 |
| | Louisiana State Dept of Hlth & Hospitals | LA | 289,273 |
| | NC State Dept/Hlth & Human Services | NC | 281,894 |
| | Maine State Dept/Health/Human Servs | ME | 273,410 |
| | NH State Dept of Health And Human Sers | NH | 266,217 |
| | Missouri State Dept/ Health & Senior Srv | MO | 263,260 |
| | Kansas State Dept of Hlth and Environmnt | KS | 259,936 |
| | Idaho State Dept of Health and Welfare | ID | 254,056 |
| | Virginia State Dept of Health | VA | 251,035 |

| Announcements (2) | Recipient | State | Award (dollars) |
|---|---|---|---|
| | Michigan State Dept of Community Health | MI | 243,670 |
| | Hawaii State Department of Health | HI | 240,142 |
| | Oklahoma State Department of Health | OK | 232,165 |
| | Maryland State Dept of Hlth/Mtl Hygiene | MD | 231,600 |
| | South Carolina State Dept of Hlth/Env | SC | 231,176 |
| | Georgia Department of Community Health | GA | 223,117 |
| | Vermont Department of Health | VT | 219,273 |
| | Oregon State Public Health Division | OR | 212,318 |
| | City of Philadelphia Public Health Dept | PA | 183,688 |
| | Pennsylvania State Dept of Health | PA | 166,089 |
| | Wyoming State Department of Health | WY | 163,444 |
| | Puerto Rico Department of Health | PR | 156,230 |
| | Nebraska St Dept of Health & Human Servs | NE | 148,500 |
| | Connecticut State Dept of Public Health | CT | 145,694 |
| | South Dakota State Dept of Health | SD | 145,267 |
| | North Dakota State Department of Health | ND | 138,776 |
| | City of Chicago | IL | 136,789 |
| | Arizona State Department of Hlth Srvcs | AZ | 117,120 |
| | West Virginia State Dept Hlth/Human Rscs | WV | 96,448 |
| | NV State Dept of Hlth/Human Svcs | NV | 90,000 |
| | Houston City Health & Human Services | TX | 89,443 |
| | Republic of Palau Ministry of Health | PW | 84,773 |
| | DC Department of Health | DC | 10,000 |
| | **Total (58 awards)** | | **$16,700,000** |
| 2. Patient Protection and Affordable Care Act (PPACA); Emerging Infections Program (EIP); Enhancing Epidemiology and Laboratory Capacity (U01) (RFA-CI-10-003)<br><br>**Purpose (award type)**: To support state and local health departments' surveillance infrastructure through enhancement of the epidemiology and laboratory capacity of the existing Emerging Infections Program network. (New) | Minnesota State Dept Of Health | MN | $322,544 |
| | Georgia Department of Community Health | GA | 309,358 |
| | Colorado State Dept/Pub Hlth & Environmt | CO | 295,655 |
| | New Mexico State Department of Health | NM | 256,398 |
| | Oregon State Public Health Division | OR | 255,704 |
| | Connecticut State Dept of Public Health | CT | 247,028 |
| | Maryland State Dept of Hlth/Mtl Hygiene | MD | 230,728 |
| | New York State Dept of Health | NY | 202,009 |
| | California Department of Public Health | CA | 198,869 |
| | Tennessee State Department of Health | TN | 181,707 |

| Announcements (2) | Recipient | State | Award (dollars) |
|---|---|---|---|
| **Legislative Authority**: Sections 301(a) [42 U.S.C. 241(a)] and 317(k) (2) [42 U.S.C. 247b (k) (2)] of the Public Health Service Act, as amended and the Patient Protection and Affordable Care Act (PPACA) of 2010 (Public Law 111-148).<br><br>**Eligibility**: Limited to ten state health departments or their bona fide agents also funded through the Emerging Infections Program funding announcements CI02-174 and CI05-026 in order to build upon the existing Emerging Infections Program infrastructure, capabilities, and activities. | **Total (10 awards)** | | **$2,500,000** |

Source: GAO analysis of HHS information.

**Table 26: FY 2011 Grants, Epidemiology and Laboratory Capacity Grants**

| Announcements (2) | Recipient | State | Award (dollars) |
|---|---|---|---|
| 1. Patient Protection and Affordable Care Act Epidemiology and Laboratory Capacity for Infectious Diseases Building and Strengthening Epidemiology, Laboratory and Health Information Systems Capacity in State and Local Health Departments (CDC-RFA-CI10–101202PPHF11) | Iowa State Dept of Public Health | IA | $1,553,629 |
| | Utah State Department of Health | UT | 1,483,303 |
| | New York City Health/Mental Hygiene | NY | 1,342,974 |
| | Indiana State Department of Health | IN | 1,250,965 |
| **Purpose (award type)**: To enhance public health programs to improve health and help restrain the rate of growth of health care costs through building epidemiology, laboratory, and health information systems capacity in state and local public health departments. (Continuation) | Michigan State Dept of Community Health | MI | 1,088,593 |
| | Massachusetts State Dept of Pub Health | MA | 1,073,121 |
| | Wisconsin Department of Health Services | WI | 1,053,518 |
| | NC State Dept/Hlth & Human Services | NC | 1,015,354 |
| | Alabama State Dept of Public Health | AL | 987,592 |
| **Legislative Authority**: Public Health Service Act Sections 301(a) [42 U.S.C. 241(a)] and 317(k) (2) [42 U.S.C. 247b (k) (2)], as amended and the Patient Protection and Affordable Care Act (PL 111-148), Title IV, Sections 4002 and 4304 (Prevention and Public Health Fund). | Houston City Health & Human Services | TX | 930,520 |
| | Alaska State Department of Hlth-Soc Svcs | AK | 927,070 |
| | Texas State Dept of Health Services | TX | 904,754 |
| | West Virginia State Dept Hlth/Human Rscs | WV | 901,911 |
| **Eligibility**: Limited to 58 state and local public health departments (or their established bona fide agents) that were 2010 grantees of Epidemiology and Laboratory Capacity for Infectious Diseases CI10-1012 funding announcement. | Minnesota State Dept of Health | MN | 860,220 |
| | Florida State Department of Health | FL | 814,429 |
| | IL State Dept of Public Health | IL | 744,130 |
| | New Mexico State Department of Health | NM | 739,137 |
| | Los Angeles County Health Services Dept | CA | 727,894 |
| | Colorado State Dept/Pub Hlth & Environmt | CO | 725,559 |
| | Virginia State Dept of Health | VA | 694,767 |
| | Maine State Dept/Health/Human Servs | ME | 692,911 |
| | Rhode Island State Dept of Health | RI | 666,375 |
| | Washington State Department of Health | WA | 663,520 |
| | NH State Dept of Health and Human Sers | NH | 654,040 |
| | Georgia Department of Community Health | GA | 636,979 |
| | Kansas State Dept of Hlth and Environmnt | KS | 633,447 |
| | Nebraska St Dept of Health & Human Servs | NE | 622,123 |
| | Ohio State Department of Health | OH | 617,083 |
| | Vermont Department of Health | VT | 602,431 |
| | Arkansas State Dept of Health | AR | 575,549 |
| | Tennessee State Department of Health | TN | 570,146 |
| | Mississippi State Department of Health | MS | 558,601 |
| | KY Cabinet for Health and Family Services | KY | 540,272 |
| | New Jersey State Dept/Health/Senior Srvs | NJ | 507,324 |
| | NY State Dept of Health | NY | 487,947 |

| Announcements (2) | Recipient | State | Award (dollars) |
|---|---|---|---|
| | MT State Dept/Pub Hlth & Human Srvs | MT | 462,058 |
| | NV State Dept of Hlth/Human Svcs | NV | 461,153 |
| | South Caronia State Dept of Hlth/Env | SC | 459,589 |
| | South Dakota State Dept of Health | SD | 444,845 |
| | Maryland State Dept of Hlth/Mtl Hygiene | MD | 441,204 |
| | Delaware State Dept of Hlth & Soc Srvs | DE | 427,619 |
| | Arizona State Department of Hlth Srvcs | AZ | 422,586 |
| | Oregon State Public Health Division | OR | 414,936 |
| | Connecticut State Dept of Public Health | CT | 406,836 |
| | Louisiana State Dept of Hlth & Hospitals | LA | 398,630 |
| | City of Philadelphia Public Health Dept | PA | 355,230 |
| | DC Department of Health | DC | 346,006 |
| | Oklahoma State Department of Health | OK | 295,015 |
| | Puerto Rico Department of Health | PR | 294,511 |
| | Missouri State Dept/ Health & Senior Srv | MO | 291,326 |
| | Wyoming State Department of Health | WY | 229,436 |
| | Idaho State Dept of Health and Welfare | ID | 228,448 |
| | CA Department of Public Health | CA | 156,034 |
| | Pennsylvania State Dept of Health | PA | 159,835 |
| | North Dakota State Department of Health | ND | 108,848 |
| | Republic of Palau Ministry of Health | PW | 69,283 |
| | Hawaii State Department of Health | HI | 40,000 |
| | City of Chicago | IL | 38,383 |
| | **Total (58 awards)** | | **$35,799,999** |
| 2. Patient Protection and Affordable Care Act, Emerging Infections Programs, Enhancing Epidemiology and Laboratory Capacity (CDC-RFA-CI10-00302PPHF11) | Minnesota State Dept of Health | MN | $313,593 |
| | Tennessee State Department of Health | TN | 307,413 |
| | New York State Dept of Health | NY | 300,477 |
| **Purpose (award type)**: To support state and local health departments' surveillance infrastructure through enhancement of the epidemiology and laboratory capacity of the existing EIP network. (Continuation) | Connecticut State Dept of Public Health | CT | 296,877 |
| | Oregon State Public Health Division | OR | 268,693 |
| | New Mexico State Department of Health | NM | 254,826 |
| **Legislative Authority**: Public Health Service Act Sections 301(a) [42 U.S.C. 241(a)] and 317(k) (2) [42 U.S.C. 247b (k) (2)], as amended and the Patient Protection and Affordable Care Act (PPACA) (Public Law 111-148), Title IV, Sections 4002 and 4304 (Prevention and Public Health Fund). | Maryland State Dept of Hlth/Mtl Hygiene | MD | 239,195 |
| | Georgia Department of Community Health | GA | 235,911 |
| | Public Health Foundation Enterprises, Inc | CA | 216,149 |
| | Colorado State Dept/Pub Hlth & Environmt | CO | 166,864 |
| **Eligibility**: Limited to state health department (or their bona fide agents) grantees funded under funding announcement CI10-003. | **Total (10 awards)** | | **$2,599,998** |

Source: GAO analysis of HHS information.

**Table 27: FY 2011 Contracts, Epidemiology and Laboratory Capacity Grants**

| Recipient | Purpose | State | Award (dollars) |
|---|---|---|---|
| Booz Allen Hamilton Inc. | CDC Program Oversight & Implementation | GA | $1,400,000 |
| Deloitte Consulting, LLP | CDC Program Oversight & Implementation | GA | 200,000 |
| **Total (2 awards)** | | | **$1,600,000** |

Source: GAO analysis of HHS information.

**Activity**: Coordinated Chronic Disease Prevention Program

The purpose of this activity is to establish or strengthen Chronic Disease
Prevention and Health Promotion programs within state health
departments, to provide leadership and coordination, support
development, implementation, and evaluation of CDC funded Chronic
Disease and Health Promotion programs. The focus is on the top five
leading chronic disease causes of death and disability (i.e., heart disease,
cancer, stroke, diabetes, and arthritis) and their associated risk factors.

- **Fiscal year 2010**: None

- **Fiscal year 2011**: $51.5 million (75 grants in three funding
  announcements totaling $49.8 million and two contracts totaling
  $1.7 million)

**Table 28: FY 2011 Grants, Coordinated Chronic Disease Prevention Program**

| Announcements (3) | Recipient | State | Award (dollars) |
|---|---|---|---|
| 1. Prevention and Public Health Fund Coordinated Chronic Disease Prevention and Health Promotion Program (CDC-RFA-DP09-9010301PPHF11)<br><br>**Purpose (award type)**: To establish or strengthen Chronic Disease Prevention and Health Promotion Programs within State Health Departments, to provide leadership and coordination, support development, implementation and evaluation of CDC funded Chronic Disease Prevention and Health Promotion programs, focusing on the top five leading chronic disease causes of death and disability (e.g. heart disease, cancer, stroke, diabetes, and arthritis) and their associated risk factors, in order to increase efficiency and impact of categorical diseases and risk factor prevention programs, including, but not limited to heart disease, cancer prevention and control, stroke, arthritis, diabetes, nutrition, physical activity and obesity. (Supplement)<br><br>**Legislative Authority**: Sections 4002 of the Affordable Care Act and 301(a) and 317(k) (2) of the Public Health Service Act (PHS Act), 42 U.S.C. 241(a) and 247b (k)(2).<br><br>**Eligibility**: Limited to States, District of Columbia and Territorial (Puerto Rico and Virgin Islands) health departments or their Bona Fide Agent. Eligibility is also limited to grantees currently funded under DP09-901 Collaborative Chronic Disease, Health Promotion, and Surveillance Program Announcement: Tobacco Control, Diabetes Prevention and Control, and Behavioral Risk Factor Surveillance System, National Center for Chronic Disease Prevention and Health Promotion. | California Department of Public Health | CA | $1,915,243 |
| | Texas State Dept of Health Services | TX | 1,509,549 |
| | New York State Dept of Health | NY | 1,290,563 |
| | Florida State Department of Health | FL | 1,182,915 |
| | ASTDHPPHE | DC | 1,128,816 |
| | Ohio State Department of Health | OH | 933,930 |
| | Pennsylvania State Dept of Health | PA | 930,987 |
| | NC State Dept/Hlth & Human Services | NC | 911,104 |
| | Georgia Department of Community Health | GA | 898,871 |
| | Michigan State Dept of Community Health | MI | 883,445 |
| | Arizona State Department of Hlth Srvcs | AZ | 842,629 |
| | Missouri State Dept/ Health & Senior Srv | MO | 784,312 |
| | Mississippi State Department of Health | MS | 778,962 |
| | Illinois State Dept of Public Health | IL | 778,232 |
| | Tennessee State Department of Health | TN | 775,664 |
| | Louisiana State Dept of Hlth & Hospitals | LA | 763,822 |
| | Virginia State Dept of Health | VA | 763,407 |
| | Massachusetts State Dept of Pub Health | MA | 757,121 |
| | New Jersey State Dept/Health/Senior Srvs | NJ | 748,849 |
| | KY Cabinet For Health and Family Services | KY | 748,295 |
| | Washington State Department of Health | WA | 748,177 |
| | Alabama State Dept of Public Health | AL | 715,499 |
| | Wisconsin Department of Health Services | WI | 697,830 |
| | South Carolina State Dept of Hlth/Env | SC | 690,357 |
| | Oklahoma State Department of Health | OK | 682,853 |
| | Oregon State Public Health Division | OR | 682,598 |
| | Maryland State Dept of Hlth/Mtl Hygiene | MD | 673,446 |
| | Arkansas State Dept of Health | AR | 672,980 |
| | Colorado State Dept/Pub Hlth & Environmt | CO | 672,949 |
| | New Mexico State Department of Health | NM | 665,704 |
| | Minnesota State Dept of Health | MN | 651,463 |
| | Kansas State Dept of Hlth And Environmnt | KS | 639,334 |
| | DC Department of Health | DC | 626,219 |
| | Indiana State Department of Health | IN | 600,000 |
| | Iowa State Dept of Public Health | IA | 600,000 |

| Announcements (3) | Recipient | State | Award (dollars) |
|---|---|---|---|
| | West Virginia State Dept Hlth/Human Rscs | WV | 600,000 |
| | Nevada State Dept of Hlth/Human Svcs | NV | 583,865 |
| | Connecticut State Dept of Public Health | CT | 569,287 |
| | Rhode Island State Dept of Health | RI | 559,000 |
| | Montana State Dept/Pub Hlth & Human Srvs | MT | 554,321 |
| | Utah State Department of Health | UT | 552,360 |
| | Maine State Dept/Health/Human Servs | ME | 551,920 |
| | Nebraska St Dept of Health & Human Servs | NE | 534,440 |
| | Idaho State Dept of Health And Welfare | ID | 530,612 |
| | Delaware State Dept of Hlth & Soc Srvs | DE | 505,981 |
| | North Dakota State Department of Health | ND | 502,238 |
| | Puerto Rico Department of Health | PR | 491,271 |
| | Vermont Department of Health | VT | 479,632 |
| | Alaska State Department of Hlth-Soc Svcs | AK | 479,112 |
| | NH State Dept of Health and Human Sers | NH | 463,729 |
| | South Dakota State Dept of Health | SD | 453,480 |
| | Hawaii State Department of Health | HI | 445,130 |
| | Wyoming State Department of Health | WY | 411,507 |
| | **Total (53 awards)** | | **$38,614,010** |
| 2. Prevention and Public Health Fund Pacific Islands Coordinated Chronic Disease Prevention and Health Promotion Program (CDC-RFA-DP09-9020303PPHF-11) | Guam Department of Public Health-Soc Svc | GU | $213,280 |
| | American Samoa Department of Health | AS | 204,846 |
| | Federated States Micronesia | FM | 207,868 |
| | Republic/Marshall Island Mnstry of Hlth | MH | 204,836 |
| | Commonwealth N Mariana Is Dept Pub Hlth | MP | 203,745 |
| | Republic of Palau Ministry of Health | PW | 199,599 |
| | **Total (6 awards)** | | **$1,234,174** |

**Purpose (award type)**: To establish or strengthen Chronic Disease Prevention and Health Promotion Programs within Territory Health Departments, to provide leadership and coordination, support development, implementation and evaluation of CDC funded Chronic Disease Prevention and Health Promotion programs, focusing on the top five leading chronic disease causes of death and disability (e.g. heart disease, cancer, stroke, diabetes, and arthritis) and their associated risk factors, in order to increase efficiency and impact of categorical diseases and risk factor prevention programs, including, but not limited to heart disease, cancer prevention and control, stroke, arthritis, diabetes, nutrition, physical activity and obesity. (Supplement)

**Legislative Authority**: Sections 4002 of the Affordable Care Act and 301(a) and 317(k) (2) of the Public Health Service Act (PHS Act), 42 U.S.C. 241(a) and 247b (k)(2).

| Announcements (3) | Recipient | State | Award (dollars) |
|---|---|---|---|
| **Eligibility**: Limited to health departments of U.S. Territories or their Bona Fide Agent, American Samoa, Federated States of Micronesia, Guam, Marshall Islands, Palau and Northern Mariana Islands. Eligibility is also limited to Grantees currently funded under DP09-902 Affiliated Pacific Island Collaborative Performance Agreement. | | | |
| 3.  Nutrition, Physical Activity and Obesity Program (CDC-RFA-DP08-805)<br><br>**Purpose (award type)**: To improve healthful eating and physical activity to prevent and control obesity and other chronic diseases by building and sustaining statewide capacity, and implementing population based strategies and interventions. (New)<br><br>**Legislative Authority**: Section 317 (k)(2) of the Public Health Service Act, [42 U.S.C. section 247b(k)(2), as amended].<br><br>**Eligibility**: State health departments and their bona fide agents (this includes the District of Columbia, the Commonwealth of Puerto Rico, the Virgin Islands, the Commonwealth of the Northern Mariana Islands, American Samoa, Guam, the Federated States of Micronesia, the Republic of the Marshall Islands, and the Republic of Palau). | Massachusetts State Dept of Pub Health | MA | $900,137 |
| | Washington State Department of Health | WA | 842,927 |
| | Iowa State Dept of Public Health | IA | 782,031 |
| | Rhode Island State Dept of Health | RI | 735,819 |
| | New Jersey State Dept/Health/Senior Srvs | NJ | 726,377 |
| | South Carolina State Dept of Hlth/Env | SC | 695,145 |
| | Wisconsin Department of Health Services | WI | 683,659 |
| | California Department of Public Health | CA | 657,358 |
| | Nebraska St Dept of Health & Human Servs | NE | 653,178 |
| | Texas State Dept of Health Services | TX | 631,161 |
| | Georgia Department of Community Health | GA | 597,369 |
| | Arizona State Dept of Health | AR | 579,957 |
| | NH State Dept of Health and Human Sers | NH | 445,500 |
| | Utah State Department of Health | UT | 416,324 |
| | Tennessee State Department of Health | TN | 335,754 |
| | Indiana State Department of Health | IN | 317,304 |
| | **Total (16 awards)** | | **$10,000,000** |

Source: GAO analysis of HHS information.

**Table 29: FY 2011 Contracts, Coordinated Chronic Disease Prevention Program**

| Recipient | Purpose | State | Award (dollars) |
|---|---|---|---|
| Four Seasons Environmental | CDC Program Oversight & Implementation | GA | $1,490,000 |
| Deloitte Consulting | CDC Program Oversight & Implementation | GA | 200,000 |
| Total (2 awards) | | | $1,690,000 |

Source: GAO analysis of HHS information.

<u>Activity</u>: CDC Healthcare Surveillance and Statistics

The purpose of this activity is to support the efforts of CDC programs including: Health Information Exchange, Enhancing Healthcare Data Access and Use and Health Service Research Capacity, National Health and Nutrition Examination Survey, Public Health Surveillance Program Office—National Center for Health Statistics Centers for Medicare and Medicaid Services Data Project, National Health Interview Survey, National Youth Fitness Survey, and Behavioral Risk Factor Surveillance System.

- **Fiscal year 2010**: $19.4 million (two grants in two funding announcements totaling $0.7 million and 12 contracts totaling $18.7 million)

- **Fiscal year 2011**: $29.5 million (13 contracts)

**Table 30: FY 2010 Grants, CDC Healthcare Surveillance and Statistics**

| Announcements (2) | Recipient | State | Award (dollars) |
|---|---|---|---|
| 1. American Recovery and Reinvestment Act of 2009: Communities Putting Prevention to Work (CDC-RFA-DP09-912ARRA09) | Arkansas State Dept of Health | AR | $200,770 |
| | Total (1 award) | | $200,770 |

**Purpose (award type)**: To create healthier communities through sustainable, proven, population-based approaches such as broad-based policy, systems, organizational and environmental changes in communities and schools. (New)

**Legislative Authority**: Section 311 and 317(k)(2) of the Public Health Service Act, 42 U.S. Code 243 and 247b(k)2.

**Eligibility**: State and local health departments or bona fide agencies, federally recognized tribal governments, regional area Indian health boards, urban Indian organizations, and inter-tribal councils. For this funding announcement, the term "states" includes the 50 states, the Commonwealth of Puerto Rico, the Virgin Islands, and the Commonwealth of the Northern Mariana Islands, American Samoa, Guam, the Federated States of Micronesia, the Republic of the Marshall Islands, and the Republic of Palau.

| Announcements (2) | Recipient | State | Award (dollars) |
|---|---|---|---|
| 2. Cancer Prevention and Control Activities (CDC-RFA-DP08-814) | American Cancer Society | GA | $499,582 |
| | Total (1 award) | | $499,582 |

**Purpose (award type)**: To assist with developing and disseminating current national, state, and community-based comprehensive information on cancer prevention, early detection, diagnosis, treatment, and survivorship; developing and disseminating professional education programs; promoting the analysis and development of evaluation, surveillance and research data, and its translation into public health messages, practice and programs; and, facilitating the exchange of expertise and coordination of programmatic efforts related to cancer prevention and control among a variety of public, private, and not-for-profit agencies at the national, state, tribal, territory and community level. (New)

**Legislative Authority**: Sections 301(a), 317(k)(2) of the Public Health Service Act, [42 U.S.C. 241(a) and 247b(k)(2)], as amended.

**Eligibility**: National public and private nonprofit organizations and faith based organizations.

Source: GAO analysis of HHS information.

**Table 31: FY 2010 Contracts, CDC Healthcare Surveillance and Statistics**

| Recipient | Purpose | State | Award (dollars) |
|---|---|---|---|
| US Census Bureau | Enhancing National Ambulatory Medical Care Survey (NAMCS) and National Hospital Ambulatory Medical Care Survey (NHAMCS) data on preventive services through computerized collection of NAMCS and NHAMCS data through induction interviews for providers. | MD | $5,782,500 |
| US Census Bureau | Enhancing National Ambulatory Medical Care Survey (NAMCS) and National Hospital Ambulatory Medical Care Survey (NHAMCS) data on preventive services through computerized collection of NAMCS and NHAMCS data through induction interviews for providers. | MD | 4,053,529 |
| US Census Bureau | Conduct the National Health Interview Survey 2010 through data collection of approximately 64,000 assigned households using trained National Health Interview Survey field representatives. | MD | 2,975,000 |
| SciMetricka | Demonstrating public health utility of health data sources through a 2-yr research study to establish utility of healthcare surveillance purposes of alternative health data sources | GA | 1,976,536 |
| Agilex Technologies | Conduct a 2-year research study to estimate the relative or cumulative value of improvement in morbidity or deaths prevented by increasing the use of clinical preventive services in entire populations | GA | 850,696 |
| SciMetricka | Demonstrating public health utility of health data sources through a 2-yr research study to establish utility of healthcare surveillance purposes of alternative health data sources | GA | 745,000 |
| Buccaneer Computer Systems | Expand the analytic utility of CMS data for research at NCHS to support newly emerging health care reform priorities, and expand the availability of CMS data for tracking the provision, use, effectiveness, and impact of primary and secondary preventative healthcare services and surveillance of selected health outcomes | VA | 649,710 |
| Westat Inc. | Provide services to complete all activities required for data collection at a primary sampling unit (PSU) component of the National Health and Nutrition Examination Survey program during Partition 4 of the data collection plan. | MD | 596,000 |
| Deloitte Consulting, LLP | Business services support - Financial Management Office | GA | 499,982 |
| Global Evaluation & Applied Research Solutions | Support for National Ambulatory Medical Care Survey (NAMCS) and National Hospital Ambulatory Medical Care Survey (NHAMCS) through data programming and processing tasks in conjunction with the development, implementation, and maintenance of computerized data collection systems for NAMCS and NHAMCS in the Division of Health Care Statistics (DHCS) | GA | 296,472 |
| Global Evaluation & Applied Research Solutions | Support for National Ambulatory Medical Care Survey (NAMCS) and National Hospital Ambulatory Medical Care Survey (NHAMCS) through data programming and processing tasks in conjunction with the development, implementation, and maintenance of computerized data collection systems for NAMCS and NHAMCS in the Division of Health Care Statistics (DHCS) | GA | 217,500 |
| Deloitte Consulting, LLP | Business services support - Health Reform Implementation Office | GA | 61,235 |
| **Total (12 awards)** | | | **$18,704,160** |

Source: GAO analysis of HHS information.

**Table 32: FY 2011 Contracts, CDC Healthcare Surveillance and Statistics**

| Recipient | Purpose | State | Award (dollars) |
|---|---|---|---|
| US Census Bureau, Demographic Surveys Division | NHIS Healthcare Reform Monitoring | GA | $10,900,000 |
| US Census Bureau | Support Services for the National Health Care Surveys – Census | MD | 10,571,195 |
| Agilex Technologies, Inc. | States, Communities, and Health Information Exchanges for Prevention and Public Health | GA | 2,789,133 |
| Research Triangle Institute | Leveraging Beacon Communities' Experience in Health Information Exchange for Public and Population Health | GA | 1,417,390 |
| Goodwill Industries of North Georgia | CDC Program Oversight & Implementation | GA | 1,050,000 |
| Johns Hopkins University Applied Physics Laboratory | Enhancing Healthcare Data Access and Use and Health Service Research Capacity | GA | 598,523 |
| Global Evaluation & Applied Research Solutions (GEARS) | Support Services for the National Health Care Surveys – GEARS | MD | 531,795 |
| International Society for Disease | Developing Business and Infrastructure Requirements for Syndromic Surveillance using Clinical Data from Health Information Exchanges | GA | 449,934 |
| Social & Scientific Systems, Inc. | Health Indicators Warehouse | MD | 291,000 |
| Systems Research and Applications Corporation | Support Services for the National Health Care Surveys – SRA | MD | 287,010 |
| Westat, Inc. | Trailer refurbishment | MD | 250,000 |
| Westat, Inc. | Physical Activity and Fitness Feasibility Study | MD | 240,000 |
| Deloitte Consulting, LLP | CDC Program Oversight & Implementation | GA | 150,000 |
| **Total (13 awards)** | | | **$29,525,980** |

Source: GAO analysis of HHS information.

## Activity: ARRA: Communities Putting Prevention to Work

The purpose of this activity is to address two of the leading preventable causes of death and disability, obesity and tobacco use, through the locally driven initiative Communities Putting Prevention to Work.

- **Fiscal year 2010**: $35.0 million (nine grants in one funding announcement totaling $29.0 million and eight contracts totaling $6.0 million)

- **Fiscal year 2011**: None

**Table 33: FY 2010 Grants, ARRA: Communities Putting Prevention to Work**

| Announcement | Recipients | State | Award (dollars) |
| --- | --- | --- | --- |
| American Recovery and Reinvestment Act (Recovery Act): Communities Putting Prevention to Work: State Competitive Supplemental Funding for Behavioral Risk Factor Surveillance System (CDC-RFA-DP09-90102-ARRA09) | City of Chicago | IL | $5,800,000 |
| | Pinellas County Health Dept | FL | 4,350,000 |
| | Southern Nevada Health District | NV | 3,800,000 |
| **Purpose (award type)**: To provide state health departments with resources to collect BRFSS baseline and follow up data from communities funded under Communities Putting Prevention to Work funding announcement, CDC-RFA-DP09-912ARRA09. (Supplement) | County of Santa Clara | CA | 3,600,000 |
| | NC State Dept/Hlth & Human Services | NC | 3,200,000 |
| | Alabama State Dept of Public Health | AL | 2,500,000 |
| **Legislative Authority**: Sections 301, 307, 310, and 311 of the Public Health Service Act, as amended, and the Comprehensive Smoking Education Act of 1984, Comprehensive Smokeless Tobacco Health Education Act of 1986, and the American Recovery and Reinvestment Act of 2009 (Recovery Act) Public Law 111-5. | Dekalb County Board of Public Health | GA | 2,350,000 |
| | Arkansas State Dept of Health | AR | 1,800,000 |
| | South Carolina State Dept of Hlth/Env | SC | 1,606,981 |
| **Eligibility**: Limited to 30 state health departments and the District of Columbia that are funded under Communities Putting Prevention to Work funding announcement, CDC-RFA-DP09-912ARRA09. | **Total (9 awards)** | | **$29,006,981** |

Source: GAO analysis of HHS information.

**Table 34: FY 2010 Contracts, ARRA: Communities Putting Prevention to Work**

| Recipient | Purpose | State | Award (dollars) |
|---|---|---|---|
| MACRO | Training Resource Center for community action | GA | $2,584,665 |
| MACRO | Support multiple evaluation components of the Communities Putting Prevention to Work initiative in communities and states. | GA | 1,748,195 |
| Northrop Grumman | Software development, integration of applications, web development, and maintenance of the infrastructure to support systems. The contractor will provide systems support and studies for research activities related to public health practice and research. | GA | 500,000 |
| Research Triangle Institute | Communities Putting Prevention to Work (CPPW) is to implement supportive policies, systems, and environments that will drive changes in behaviors to reduce risk factors, prevent/delay chronic diseases, promote wellness in children and adults, and provide positive sustainable health changes in communities. | GA | 398,900 |
| McKing Consulting | Management Consultation and Technical Assistance Services in Support of the Nutrition, Physical Activity and Obesity Programs. | GA | 349,993 |
| Research Triangle Institute | To customize a system dynamic evaluation model to project the impact policy, systems, and governmental changes in the approximately 44 Communities Putting Prevention to Work (CPPW) initiative and the 8 additional communities funded through the Affordable Care Act. | GA | 195,488 |
| GMI & DESA JOINT VENTURE | Contribute to the national agenda for obesity prevention and control | GA | 190,000 |
| Northrop Grumman | Support all aspects of full lifecycle application systems development and maintenance on a variety of platforms including mainframe, client server, and web; architecture and infrastructure design to support enterprise application software services including hardware/software/network design and implementation; database design, application development and support; data management and security controls; quality assurance, test and control functions; and technical communication, consultation and information support. | GA | 9,000 |
| **Total (8 awards)** | | | **$5,976,241** |

Source: GAO analysis of HHS information.

## Activity: Environmental Public Health Tracking

The purpose of this activity is to establish and maintain a nationwide tracking network to collect, integrate, analyze, and translate health and environmental data for use in public health practice and policy development. This activity is designed to build environmental public health surveillance (tracking) capacity in additional state and local health departments by enhancing infrastructure, data, partnerships, and workforce.

- **Fiscal year 2010**: None

- **Fiscal year 2011**: $30.8 million (30 grants in five funding
  announcements totaling $22.8 million and contracts totaling
  $8.0 million)

**Table 35: FY 2011 Grants, Environmental Public Health Tracking**

| Announcements (5) | Recipient | State | Award (dollars) |
|---|---|---|---|
| 1. National Environmental Public Health Tracking Program (CDC-RFA-EH09-907)<br>2. National Environmental Public Health Tracking Program-Network Implementation (CDC-RFA-EH11-1103)<br><br>**Purpose (award type)**: To establish and maintain a nationwide tracking network to obtain integrated health and environmental data and use it to provide information in support of actions that improve the health of communities. The program also aims to build state and local public health capacity in the area of environmental health surveillance. (New and Continuation)<br><br>**Legislative Authority**: Sections 311 and 317(k)(2) of the Public Health Service Act, [42 U.S.C. Sections 243 and 247b(k)(2)] as amended.<br><br>**Eligibility**: For CDC-RFA-EH09-907, federally recognized or state-recognized American Indian/Alaska Native tribal governments, state and local governments or their Bona Fide Agents, and political subdivisions of states; and for CDC-RFA-EH11-1103, state and local government health departments, or their Bona Fide Agents, which were originally selected through a competitive award process under CDC Program Announcement CDC-RFA-EH06-601 of 2006 – National Environmental Public Health Tracking Program- Network Implementation. | Missouri State Dept/ Health & Senior Srv | MO | $1,100,000 |
| | New Mexico State Department of Health | NM | 1,100,000 |
| | Oregon State Public Health Division | OR | 1,100,000 |
| | Utah State Department of Health | UT | 1,100,000 |
| | Wisconsin Department of Health Services | WI | 1,100,000 |
| | California Department of Public Health | CA | 1,099,998 |
| | New York State Dept of Health | NY | 1,099,995 |
| | New York City Health/Mental Hygiene | NY | 1,099,894 |
| | Washington State Department of Health | WA | 1,099,121 |
| | Massachusetts State Dept of Pub Health | MA | 1,073,968 |
| | Maryland State Dept of Hlth/Mtl Hygiene | MD | 1,047,251 |
| | Maine State Dept/Health/Human Servs | ME | 1,004,719 |
| | Florida State Department of Health | FL | 963,629 |
| | Minnesota State Dept of Health | MN | 875,000 |
| | South Carolina State Dept of Hlth/Env | SC | 862,000 |
| | Pennsylvania State Dept of Health | PA | 815,858 |
| | New Jersey State Dept/Health/Senior Srvs | NJ | 795,691 |
| | Vermont Department of Health | VT | 753,411 |
| | Connecticut State Dept of Public Health | CT | 722,000 |
| | NH State Dept of Health and Human Sers | NH | 715,892 |
| | Louisiana State Dept of Hlth & Hospitals | LA | 678,510 |
| | Colorado State Dept/Pub Hlth & Environmt | CO | 656,802 |
| | Kansas State Dept of Hlth and Environmnt | KS | 577,596 |
| | Iowa State Dept of Public Health | IA | 370,273 |
| | **Total (24 awards)** | | **$21,811,608** |

| Announcements (5) | Recipient | State | Award (dollars) |
|---|---|---|---|
| 3. Non-Competitive 12-month Cost Extension Supplement for CDC-RFA-HM08-8050301SUPP10: Affordable Care Act (ACA): Capacity Building Assistance to Strengthen Public Health Infrastructure and Performance (CDC-RFA-HM08-8050401PPHF11) | Council of State and Territorial Epidemiologists | GA | $250,000 |
| | Association of State and Territorial Health Officials | VA | 235,000 |
| | National Association of City/County Health Officials | DC | 150,400 |
| **Purpose (award type)**: To support the provision of capacity building assistance to state, tribal, local and | American Public Health Association | DC | 100,000 |
| territorial health departments that ensures performance improvement and successful adoption of best or promising practices to address key areas of public health infrastructure investments. (Supplement) | **Total (4 awards)** | | **$735,400** |
| **Legislative Authority**: Sections 301 and 317 of the Public Health Service Act (PHS Act), 42 USC, 241 and 247b as amended. Funding is appropriated under the Affordable Care Act (PL 111-148), Title IV, Section 4002 (Prevention and Public Health Fund). | | | |
| **Eligibility**: Limited to specific national, non-profit, public health professional organizations funded through the competitive funding opportunity, CDC-RFA-HM08-8030301SUPP10. | | | |
| 4. National Environmental Public Health Tracking Program National Association for Health Data Organizations (CDC-RFA-EH10-1003) | Nat. Assoc. of Health Data Orgs. | UT | $124,995 |
| | **Total (1 award)** | | **$124,995** |
| **Purpose (award type)**: To continue a partnership with the National Association of Health Data Organizations. (Continuation) | | | |
| **Legislative Authority**: Section 317(k) (2) of the Public Health Service Act, [42 U.S.C Section 247b(k)(2)], as amended. | | | |
| **Eligibility**: Limited to the National Association of Health Data Organizations. | | | |
| 5. National Environmental Public Health Tracking Program National Association for Public Health Statistics and Information Systems (CDC-RFA-EH10-1004) | NAPHSIS | MD | $125,000 |
| | **Total (1 award)** | | **$125,000** |
| **Purpose (award type)**: To promote collaboration among vital records, health statistics, and health information systems professionals to provide environmental and health data information to public health practitioners, policy makers, and the public. (Continuation) | | | |
| **Legislative Authority**: Section 311 and 317 (k)(2) of the Public Health Service Act, [42 U. S. C. Section 243 and 247b(k)(2)] as amended. | | | |
| **Eligibility**: Limited to the National Association for Public Health Statistics and Information Systems. | | | |

Source: GAO analysis of HHS information.

**Table 36: FY 2011 Contracts, Environmental Public Health Tracking**

| Recipient | Purpose | State | Award (dollars) |
|---|---|---|---|
| TKC Global | IT Support - TKC Global | GA | $1,489,663 |
| Battelle | IT Support - Battelle IT | GA | 1,260,000 |
| Battelle memorial Institute | IT Support - Battelle (DM) | GA | 808,600 |
| University of California, Berkeley | Environmental Public Health Tracking Program | CA | 612,144 |
| GSA/FAS/4TRE | Information technology, data management, and support services for surveillance public health activities | GA | 574,869 |
| Healthy Housing Solutions, Inc. | Tobacco Control: Adoption, Health Impact | GA | 399,999 |
| University of Illinois-Chicago | Environmental Public Health Tracking Program | IL | 353,354 |
| University of Medicine and Dentistry – New Jersey | Environmental Public Health Tracking Program | NJ | 297,197 |
| The Regents of The University of California | Environmental Public Health Tracking Program | CA | 292,318 |
| GSA/FAS/4TRE | Development of a Climate Change Module to track predictors, responses and public health consequences of climate | GA | 263,895 |
| NASA | Return On Investment | GA | 225,000 |
| University of Pittsburgh | Environmental Public Health Tracking Program | PA | 223,838 |
| University of Utah | Academic Partners - Schools of Public Health | UT | 221,721 |
| University of Pittsburgh | Environmental Public Health Tracking Program | PA | 197,022 |
| Booz Allen Hamilton Inc. | GRASP | GA | 185,000 |
| GSA/FAS/4TRE | Air Pollution and Respiratory Health Branch National Asthma Control Program Workgroups | GA | 154,225 |
| SMITHKLINE BEECHAM CORPORATION | Environmental Tracking | GA | 153,607 |
| Emory University | Field Test/Training Exercise | GA | 146,394 |
| PRR, Inc. | Health Marketing Communication | GA | 96,075 |
| Various - Emory University, JP Morgan Chase, Northrop Grumman | Contracts <$25K | GA | 65,101 |
| **Total** | | | **$8,020,022** |

Source: GAO analysis of HHS information.

## Activity: Public Health Workforce

The purpose of this activity is to help ensure a prepared, diverse, sustainable public health workforce. PPHF funding leverages critical workforce development activities supported with CDC's core budget.

- **Fiscal year 2010**: $ 4.7 million (four grants in one funding
  announcement totaling $0.8 million and 17 contracts totaling
  $3.8 million)

- **Fiscal year 2011**: $18.5 million (four grants in two funding
  announcements totaling $4.7 million and 27 contracts totaling
  $13.8 million)

**Table 37: FY 2010 Grants, Public Health Workforce**

| Announcement | Recipient | State | Award (dollars) |
|---|---|---|---|
| Competitive Supplement to CDC-RFA-HM08-805: Strengthen and Improve the Nation's Capacity through National, Non-profit, Professional Public Health Organizations to Increase Health Protection and Health Equity (CDC-RFA-HM08-8050301SUPP10) | Council of State and Territorial Epidemiologists | GA | $335,000 |
| | Dekalb County Board of Public Health | GA | 250,000 |
| | Public Health Foundation | DC | 172,000 |
| | Association of State and Territorial Health Officials | VA | 75,000 |
| **Purpose (award type)**: To support the provision of capacity building assistance to state, tribal, local and territorial health departments that ensures successful adoption of best or promising practices to address key areas of public health infrastructure investments. (Supplement) | **Total (4 awards)** | | **$832,000** |

**Legislative Authority**: Sections 301 and 317 of the
Public Health Service Act (PHS Act), 42 USC, 241
and 247b as amended. Funding is appropriated
under the Affordable Care Act (PL 111-148), Title IV,
Section 4002 (Prevention and Public Health Fund).

**Eligibility**: Limited to national, non-profit, and public
health professional organizations funded through the
competitive funding announcement
CDC-RFA-HM08-805.

Source: GAO analysis of HHS information.

GAO-12-788 Prevention and Public Health Fund

**Table 38: FY 2010 Contracts, Public Health Workforce**

| Recipient | Purpose | State | Award (dollars) |
|---|---|---|---|
| Office of Personnal Management | PHAP Management & Operations Support | GA | $1,700,860 |
| Deloitte Consulting, LLP | Evaluation/Education/Curriculum Development (All Fellowships) | GA | 912,705 |
| Chickasaw Adv | IT/informatics Nees/EIS Secure Website | GA | 264,220 |
| Deloitte Consulting, LLP | Evaluation/Education/Curriculum Development (All Fellowships) | GA | 199,605 |
| Chickasaw Adv | Sr. Health Communication Specialist | GA | 118,694 |
| Chickasaw Adv | Public Health Analyst (All Fellowships) | GA | 116,274 |
| Chickasaw Adv | Public Health Advisor (PHPS) | GA | 107,192 |
| Annual EIS Conference Support | Administrative and Logistical Support to the Public Health Apprentice Program | GA | 70,000 |
| Chickasaw Adv | Health Comm Specialist I (All Fellowships) | GA | 56,371 |
| Chickasaw Adv | Web Developer I (All Fellowships) | GA | 54,428 |
| Midtown Personnel | Administrative Assistant III (PHPS) | GA | 42,148 |
| Emory University | Public Health Instructor | GA | 39,798 |
| Chickasaw Adv | Health Comm Specialist I (All Fellowships) | GA | 37,079 |
| Chickasaw Adv | Health Comm Specialist II (All Fellowships) | GA | 35,015 |
| Deloitte Consulting, LLP | Business services support - Health Reform Implementation Office | GA | 30,000 |
| Deloitte Consulting, LLP | Web Developer II (All Fellowships) | GA | 29,530 |
| Chickasaw Adv | Program Assistant (EIS) | GA | 14,564 |
| **Total (17 awards)** | | | **$3,828,483** |

Source: GAO analysis of HHS information.

**Table 39: FY 2011 Grants, Public Health Workforce**

| Announcements (2) | Recipient | State | Award (dollars) |
|---|---|---|---|
| 1. Association of Public Health Laboratories Cooperative Agreement (CDC-RFA-HM10-1001) | Association of Public Health Laboratories | MD | $1,000,000 |
| | **Total (1 award)** | | **$1,000,000** |
| **Purpose (award type)**: To enhance the work of public health laboratories in the U.S. and abroad, to promote quality public health laboratory practice, improve public health laboratory infrastructure, strengthen the public health laboratory system, and to develop a well-trained public health laboratory workforce in the U.S. and globally. Also, to ensure laboratory preparedness for emerging infectious diseases or other biologic and chemical public health threats, promote technology transfer to ensure up-to-date technologies for the testing laboratory, and enhance communication linkages between state and local public health laboratories and the clinical laboratory testing community. (New) | | | |
| **Legislative Authority**: Sections 307 and 317(k)(2) of the Public Health Service Act, [42 U.S.C. 242l and 247b (k)(2), as amended]. | | | |
| **Eligibility**: Limited to the Association of Public Health Laboratories. | | | |
| 2. Non-Competitive 12-month Cost Extension Supplement for CDC-RFA-HM08-8050301SUPP10: Affordable Care Act (ACA): Capacity Building Assistance to Strengthen Public Health Infrastructure and Performance (CDC-RFA-HM08-8050401PPHF11) and Competitive Program Expansion Supplement for CDC-RFA-HM08-805: Strengthen and Improve the Nation's Capacity through National, Non-profit, Professional Public Health Organizations to Increase Health Protection and Health Equity (CDC-RFA-HM08-8050402PHFF11) | Council of State And Territorial Epidemiologists | GA | $3,096,706 |
| | Association of State and Territorial Health Officials | VA | 412,920 |
| | Public Health Foundation | DC | 172,000 |
| | **Total (3 awards)** | | **$3,681,626** |
| **Purpose (award type)**: To support the provision of capacity building assistance to state, tribal, local and territorial health departments that ensures performance improvement and successful adoption of best or promising practices to address key areas of public health infrastructure investments. (Supplement) | | | |
| **Legislative Authority**: Sections 301 and 317 of the Public Health Service Act (PHS Act), 42 USC, 241 and 247b as amended. Funding is appropriated under the Affordable Care Act (PL 111-148), (Prevention and Public Health Fund). | | | |
| **Eligibility**: Limited to specific national, non-profit, public health professional organizations also funded through the funding opportunity CDC-RFA-HM08-80301SUPP10 and the competitive funding opportunityCDC-RFA-HM08-805. | | | |

Source: GAO analysis of HHS information.

**Table 40: FY 2011 Contracts, Public Health Workforce**

| Recipient | Purpose | State | Award (dollars) |
|---|---|---|---|
| Scimetrika, LLC | PHPS Field Residency and Expanded Training | GA | $2,531,027 |
| Emory University Southeastern Institute for Training and Evaluation | Program Management Support – OPM IAA Strategic Human Resource Planning and Implementation to Improve Human Capital and Enterprise | GA | 2,357,192 |
| Scimetrika, LLC | Post EIS Practicum (PEP) | GA | 1,759,097 |
| Deloitte Consulting LLP | Education and Evaluation Consultation for SEPDPO Fellowship Programs | GA | 1,641,587 |
| Deloitte Consulting LLP | Fellowship Management System | GA | 1,361,629 |
| Emergint Technologies, Inc. | IT Support for SEPDPO | GA | 766,612 |
| Chickasaw Advisory Services, LLC | E Learning Expansion (Training, Education and Communication Support) | GA | 739,599 |
| Booz Allen Hamilton Inc. | CDC Program Oversight & Implementation | GA | 500,000 |
| Deloitte Consulting, LLP | CIMS Task Order Fellowship Management System | GA | 205,000 |
| DB Consulting Group, Inc. | Workforce Enumeration Project | GA | 197,222 |
| Chickasaw Advisory Services, LLC | Contractor for Informatician Job Classification Project | GA | 148,845 |
| Emergint Technologies, Inc. | Online Learning Development | GA | 142,196 |
| Chickasaw Advisory Services, LLC | Management Analyst | GA | 134,880 |
| Total Solutions, Inc. | Administrative Assistant | GA | 126,917 |
| Chickasaw Advisory Services, LLC | Web Developer/Master II | GA | 124,937 |
| Chickasaw Advisory Services, LLC | Half-time Health Communication Specialist II (1/2 time) (SW) | GA | 124,937 |
| Dell Services Federal Government, Inc. | IT Support | GA | 120,000 |
| Chickasaw Advisory Services, LLC | Web Developer | GA | 116,858 |
| Chickasaw Advisory Services, LLC | Health Communication Specialist I (MPR) | GA | 116,758 |
| Chickasaw Advisory Services, LLC | Health Communication Specialist I (SN) | GA | 112,781 |
| Chickasaw Advisory Services, LLC | Public Health Advisor | GA | 111,165 |
| Chalk And Wire | Commercial software for assessment of learning outcome (COTS Portfolio) | GA | 82,915 |
| Corporate Temps Inc | Administrative Assistant II | GA | 79,738 |
| Chickasaw Advisory Services, LLC | Program Assistant | GA | 78,519 |
| Chickasaw Advisory Services, LLC | Half-time Health Communication Specialist II | GA | 62,452 |
| Ashlin Management Group, Inc. | Tech Support for SEPDPO | GA | 28,954 |
| Professional and Scientific Associates, Inc. | PSA Training Order - Emory University Southeastern Institute for Training and Evaluation | GA | 24,631 |
| **Total (27 awards)** | | | **$13,796,447** |

Source: GAO analysis of HHS information.

## Activity: HIV/AIDS

The purpose of this activity is to support demonstration projects to identify and implement a "combination approach" to enhance effective HIV prevention programming in hard-hit areas across the country. These efforts are designed to both supplement existing programs in these communities and help jurisdictions to better focus efforts on key at-risk populations and fulfill unmet needs.

- **Fiscal year 2010**: $ 29.2 million (88 grants in three funding announcements totaling $21.6 million and six contracts totaling $7.6 million)

- **Fiscal year 2011**: None

**Table 41: FY 2010 Grants, HIV/AIDS**

| Announcements (3) | Recipient | State | Award (dollars) |
|---|---|---|---|
| 1.  HIV/AIDS Surveillance: Enhancing Laboratory Reporting (CDC-RFA-PS08-8020302SUPP10)<br>**Purpose (award type)**: To enable state and local health departments to improve the reporting of HIV laboratory data from private and public laboratories to state and local health departments and CDC. (Supplement)<br>**Legislative Authority**: Sections 317 and 318B of the Public Health Service Act (42 U.S.C. Sections 247b and 247c-2), as amended and the Patient Protection and Affordable Care Act (PL 111-148), Title IV, Section 4002 (Prevention and Public Health Fund).<br>**Eligibility**: Limited to state and local territorial health departments that are currently grantees under the funding announcement PS08-802, HIV/AIDS Surveillance. | California Department of Public Health | CA | $415,593 |
| | Florida State Department of Health | FL | 400,000 |
| | New York City Health/Mental Hygiene | NY | 393,380 |
| | New York State Dept of Health | NY | 307,033 |
| | Maryland State Dept of Hlth/Mtl Hygiene | MD | 229,857 |
| | Virginia State Dept of Health | VA | 200,000 |
| | Los Angeles County Health Services Dept | CA | 190,581 |
| | Houston City Health & Human Services | TX | 184,076 |
| | DC Department of Health | DC | 183,595 |
| | San Francisco Dept of Public Health | CA | 171,081 |
| | New Jersey State Dept/Health/Senior Srvs | NJ | 169,050 |
| | Texas State Dept of Health Services | TX | 142,681 |
| | Alabama State Dept of Public Health | AL | 136,711 |
| | City of Philadelphia Public Health Dept | PA | 136,330 |
| | Michigan State Dept of Community Health | MI | 135,438 |
| | Oklahoma State Department of Health | OK | 122,817 |
| | Minnesota State Dept of Health | MN | 117,953 |
| | Arkansas State Dept of Health | AR | 114,182 |
| | Washington State Department of Health | WA | 104,993 |
| | Utah State Department of Health | UT | 104,114 |
| | Iowa State Dept of Public Health | IA | 101,668 |
| | Louisiana State Dept of Hlth & Hospitals | LA | 97,517 |

| Announcements (3) | Recipient | State | Award (dollars) |
|---|---|---|---|
| | Wisconsin Department of Health Services | WI | 96,639 |
| | Tennessee State Department of Health | TN | 93,161 |
| | Arizona State Department of Hlth Srvcs | AZ | 90,262 |
| | Massachusetts State Dept of Pub Health | MA | 89,268 |
| | South Carolina State Dept of Hlth/Env | SC | 87,900 |
| | Oregon State Public Health Division | OR | 82,180 |
| | Connecticut State Dept of Public Health | CT | 79,714 |
| | Mississippi State Department of Health | MS | 79,020 |
| | Nevada State Dept of Hlth/Human Svcs | NV | 75,576 |
| | KY Cabinet for Health and Family Services | KY | 72,899 |
| | Illinois State Dept of Public Health | IL | 72,489 |
| | Colorado State Dept/Pub Hlth & Environmt | CO | 68,390 |
| | Nebraska St Dept of Health & Human Servs | NE | 67,735 |
| | Maine State Dept/Health/Human Servs | ME | 60,000 |
| | Delaware State Dept of Hlth & Soc Srvs | DE | 51,218 |
| | Virgin Islands Department of Health | VI | 49,750 |
| | Alaska State Department of Hlth-Soc Svcs | AK | 41,909 |
| | Hawaii State Department of Health | HI | 41,848 |
| | Georgia Department of Community Health | GA | 35,431 |
| | Puerto Rico Department of Health | PR | 29,565 |
| | Guam Department of Public Health-Soc Svc | GU | 25,000 |
| | Idaho State Dept of Health And Welfare | ID | 24,658 |
| | City of Chicago | IL | 16,941 |
| | American Samoa Department of Health | AS | 9,797 |
| | **Total (46 awards)** | | **$5,600,000** |
| 2.  Expanded Human Immunodeficiency Virus (HIV) Testing for Disproportionately Affected Populations (CDC-RFA-PS10-10138) | Alabama State Dept of Public Health | AL | $145,567 |
| | Arizona State Department of Hlth Srvcs | AZ | 145,567 |
| **Purpose (award type)**: To increase HIV testing opportunities for populations disproportionately affected | California Department of Public Health | CA | 145,567 |
| by HIV; increase the proportion of HIV-infected persons | Los Angeles County Health Services Dept | CA | 145,567 |
| in these populations who are aware of their infection and are linked to appropriate services; and identify | San Francisco Dept of Public Health | CA | 145,567 |
| strategies for leveraging resources to maximize the | Connecticut State Dept of Public Health | CT | 145,567 |
| yield and sustainability of routine HIV screening | DC Department of Health | DC | 145,567 |
| programs in healthcare settings. (New) | Florida State Department of Health | FL | 145,567 |
| **Legislative Authority**: Sections 301 and 318 of the | Georgia Department of Community Health | GA | 145,567 |
| Public Health Service Act (42 U.S.C. Section 241 and 247c), as amended. | Illinois State Dept of Public Health | IL | 145,567 |

| Announcements (3) | Recipient | State | Award (dollars) |
|---|---|---|---|
| **Eligibility**: Limited to health department jurisdictions with at least 175 estimated combined AIDS diagnoses among Blacks/African Americans and Hispanics/ Latinos in 2007. | City of Chicago | IL | 145,567 |
| | Louisiana State Dept of Hlth & Hospitals | LA | 145,567 |
| | Maryland State Dept of Hlth/Mtl Hygiene | MD | 145,567 |
| | Massachusetts State Dept of Pub Health | MA | 145,567 |
| | Michigan State Dept of Community Health | MI | 145,567 |
| | Mississippi State Department of Health | MS | 145,567 |
| | Missouri State Dept/ Health & Senior Srv | MO | 145,567 |
| | New Jersey State Dept/Health/Senior Srvs | NJ | 145,567 |
| | New York State Dept of Health | NY | 145,567 |
| | New York City Health/Mental Hygiene | NY | 145,557 |
| | NC State Dept/Hlth & Human Services | NC | 145,567 |
| | Ohio State Department of Health | OH | 145,567 |
| | City of Philadelphia Public Health Dept | PA | 145,567 |
| | Hershey Milton S Medical Center | PA | 145,567 |
| | Puerto Rico Department of Health | PR | 145,567 |
| | South Carolina State Dept of Hlth/Env | SC | 145,567 |
| | Tennessee State Department of Health | TN | 145,567 |
| | Texas State Dept of Health Services | TX | 145,567 |
| | Houston City Health & Human Services | TX | 145,567 |
| | Virginia State Dept of Health | VA | 145,567 |
| | **Total (30 awards)** | | **$4,367,000** |
| 3. Enhanced Comprehensive HIV Prevention Planning and Implementation for Metropolitan Statistical Areas Most Affected by HIV/AIDS (CDC-RFA-PS10-10181)<br><br>**Purpose (award type)**: To facilitate the development and implementation of Enhanced Comprehensive HIV Prevention Plans (ECHPPs) for geographic areas most affected by the HIV epidemic in order to reduce HIV risk and incidence in those areas. (New)<br><br>**Legislative Authority**: Sections 317(k)(2) and 318 of the Public Health Service Act (42 U.S.C. Sections 247b(k)(2) and 247c), as amended, and Section 4002 of the Patient Protection and Affordable Care Act (PL 111-148).<br><br>**Eligibility**: Limited to twelve (12) state and local governments or bona fide agencies/organizations in specific Metropolitan Statistical Areas or specified Metropolitan Divisions that have the highest estimated AIDS prevalence at the end of 2007. | New York City Health/Mental Hygiene | NY | $1,581,184 |
| | Los Angeles County Health Services Dept | CA | 1,059,407 |
| | DC Department of Health | DC | 946,403 |
| | City of Chicago | IL | 927,371 |
| | Georgia Department of Community Health | GA | 913,982 |
| | Florida State Department of Health | FL | 909,315 |
| | City of Philadelphia Public Health Dept | PA | 906,024 |
| | Houston City Health & Human Services | TX | 891,108 |
| | San Francisco Dept of Public Health | CA | 887,968 |
| | Maryland State Dept of Hlth/Mtl Hygiene | MD | 878,896 |
| | Texas State Dept of Health Services | TX | 850,016 |
| | Puerto Rico Department of Health | PR | 848,326 |
| | **Total (12 awards)** | | **$11,600,000** |

Source: GAO analysis of HHS information.

**Table 42: FY 2010 Contracts, HIV/AIDS**

| Recipient | Purpose | State | Award (dollars) |
|---|---|---|---|
| Scimetrika, LLC | Comprehensive HIV Prevention through the evaluation of Enhanced Comprehensive HIV Prevention Planning and Implementation for Metropolitan Statistical Areas most affected by HIV | NC | $3,164,520 |
| Manila Consulting Group, Inc | Web-based HIV behavioral trend analysis among men who have sex with men (MSM) | VA | 3,106,740 |
| Office of Clinical and Preventive Service Indian Health Services | To utilize interagency resources to reduce the incidence and burden of HIV and other STDs and hepatitis in the AI/AN population | MD | 1,000,000 |
| Professional & Scientific Assoc | Meeting & Conference Support for Consultation meetings for grantees of PS10-10181: "Enhanced Comprehensive HIV Prevention Planning and Implementation for Metropolitan Statistical Areas Most Affected by HIV/AIDS." | VA | 203,865 |
| Professional & Scientific Assoc | Meeting & Conference support for Consultation on Monitoring of CD4 and Viral Load Test Results In The National HIV Surveillance System | GA | 109,875 |
| Northrop Grumman | Support all aspects of full lifecycle application systems development and maintenance on a variety of platforms including mainframe, client server, and web; architecture and infrastructure design to support enterprise application software services including hardware/software/network design and implementation; database design, application development and support; data management and security controls; quality assurance, test and control functions; and technical communication, consultation and information support. | GA | 40,500 |
| **Total (6 awards)** | | | **$7,625,500** |

Source: GAO analysis of HHS information.

**Activity**: Racial and Ethnic Approaches to Community Health (REACH)

The purpose of this activity is to serve as the cornerstone of CDC's efforts to eliminate racial and ethnic disparities in health. REACH supports community coalitions that design, implement, evaluate, and disseminate community-driven strategies to eliminate health disparities in key health areas, such as heart disease, diabetes, breast and cervical cancer, immunization, asthma, hepatitis B, and infant mortality.

- **Fiscal year 2010**: None

- **Fiscal year 2011**: $24.6 million (43 grants in three funding announcements totaling $24.5 million and one contract totaling $0.1 million)

**Table 43: FY 2011 Grants, Racial and Ethnic Approaches to Community Health (REACH)**

| Announcements (3) | Recipient | State | Award (dollars) |
|---|---|---|---|
| 1. Racial and Ethnic Approaches to Community Health across the US (CDC-RFA-DP07-707)<br><br>**Purpose (award type)**: To advance evidence- and practice-based programs and culturally based community practices to eliminate racial and ethnic health disparities through implementation, evaluation, and dissemination of state of the art knowledge. (New)<br><br>**Legislative Authority**: Section 301(a) and 317(k) (2) of the Public Health Service Act, 42 U.S. Code 241(a) and 247b(k)2.<br><br>**Eligibility**: Public and private nonprofit organizations; for profit organizations; small, minority women-owned businesses; universities and colleges; hospitals; community-based and faith-based organizations; American Indian/Alaska Native tribal governments and American Indian/Alaska Native tribally designated organizations; Alaska Native health corporations; Urban Indian health organizations; tribal epidemiology centers; state and local governments or their Bona Fide agents, and political subdivisions of states. | Public Health Institute | CA | $893,128 |
| | Hildalgo Medical Services | NM | 874,499 |
| | University of Colorado At Denver And Hsc | CO | 865,189 |
| | University of Illinois At Chicago | IL | 852,874 |
| | Boston Public Health Commission | MA | 850,040 |
| | Medical University of South Carolina | SC | 850,001 |
| | University of Alabama at Birmingham | AL | 850,000 |
| | University of California, Los Angeles | CA | 850,000 |
| | University of Hawaii | HI | 850,000 |
| | Genesee County Health Department | MI | 850,000 |
| | Institute for Urban Family Health | NY | 850,000 |
| | Oklahoma State Department of Health | OK | 850,000 |
| | Greater Lawrence Family Health Center, Inc | MA | 849,999 |
| | Mount Sinai School of Medicine | NY | 849,999 |
| | Orange Co. Asian and Pacific Islander Community Alliance | CA | 844,285 |
| | New York University School of Medicine | NY | 844,248 |
| | Khmer Health Advocates, Inc. | CT | 844,243 |
| | Southeast Chicago Development Commission | IL | 427,891 |
| | Seattle-King County Department of Public Health | WA | 415,391 |
| | LA Biomedical Research Institute at Harbor | CA | 415,390 |
| | Special Services for Groups | CA | 415,390 |
| | City of Chicago | IL | 415,390 |
| | Health Visions Midwest, Inc. | IN | 415,390 |
| | Center for Comm. Health, Education and Research | MA | 415,390 |
| | Eastern Band of Cherokee Indians | NC | 415,390 |
| | YMCA of Greater Cleveland | OH | 415,390 |
| | Choctaw Nation of Oklahoma | OK | 415,390 |
| | Virginia Commonwealth University | VA | 415,390 |
| | Inter-Tribal Council of MI | MI | 415,390 |
| | West Virginia State Dept Hlth/Human Rscs | WV | 415,387 |
| | University of Arizona | AZ | 412,890 |
| | Community Health Councils, Inc. | CA | 411,370 |
| | Wai'Anac District Health and Hosp. Board | HI | 402,075 |
| | To Our Children's Future With Health, Inc | PA | 400,031 |
| | YMCA of Santa Clara Valley | CA | 400,000 |

| Announcements (3) | Recipient | State | Award (dollars) |
|---|---|---|---|
| | Children's Hospital Corporation | MA | 400,000 |
| | Brooklyn Perinatal Network | NY | 400,000 |
| | Northern Arapaho Tribe | WY | 397,808 |
| | Vernon J. Harris East End Community H Center | VA | 396,052 |
| | **Total (39 awards)** | | **$23,551,300** |
| 2. Racial and Ethnic Approaches to Community Health for Communities Organized to Respond and Evaluate (REACH) (CDC-RFA-DP10-1014) | Schenectady Co. Public Health Services | NY | $199,700 |
| | **Total (1 award)** | | **$199,700** |

**Purpose (award type)**: To support local communities to strategically organize, implement and evaluate evidence-based policy, system, and environmental change interventions that eliminate racial and ethnic health disparities in chronic diseases. In addition this announcement will support the transition of communities from the analysis of intervention results to the use of these results in facilitating health equity and policy change. (New)

**Legislative Authority**: Section 301(a) and 317(k) (2) of the Public Health Service Act, 42 U.S. Code 241(a) and 247b(k)2.

**Eligibility**: With the exception of current Racial and Ethnic Approaches to Community Health for Communities grantees, eligible applicants include: nonprofit and for-profit organizations (other than small business); small, minority women-owned businesses; universities, colleges and research institutions; hospitals; community-based and faith-based organizations; American Indian/Alaska native tribal governments and American Indian/Alaska native tribally designated organizations; Alaska Native health corporations; Urban Indian health organizations; tribal epidemiology centers, state and local governments or their Bona Fide agents, and political subdivisions of states.

| Announcements (3) | Recipient | State | Award (dollars) |
|---|---|---|---|
| 3. National Organizations that Serve Minority Communities Initiative to Share Racial and Ethnic Approaches to Eliminate Health Disparities with Local Affiliates & Chapters (CDC-RFA-DP09-905) | Asian Pacific Partners For Empowerment, Advocacy And Leadership | CA | $250,000 |
| | Inter-Tribal Council of Michigan | MI | 250,000 |
| | Joint Center For Political And Economic Studies | DC | 250,000 |
| | **Total (3 awards)** | | **$750,000** |

**Purpose (award type)**: To support national minority organizations to (1) disseminate evidence-based strategies, tools and best practices to their local affiliates and chapters; and (2) to provide capacity-building technical assistance to local affiliates and chapters to address the growing health disparities among their constituents. (New)

**Legislative Authority**: Section 301(a) and 317(k) (2) of the Public Health Service Act, 42 U.S. Code 241(a) and 247b(k)(2).

**Eligibility**: Limited to established national nonprofit and Urban Indian health organizations and federally recognized American Indian/Alaska Native tribal governments that can demonstrate experience working in the health arena and specifically on issues related to health disparities.

Source: GAO analysis of HHS information.

**Table 44: FY 2011 Contract, Racial and Ethnic Approaches to Community Health (REACH)**

| Recipient | Purpose | State | Award (dollars) |
|---|---|---|---|
| Planning Professionals, LTD. | Racial and Ethnic Health Disparities Action Institute (REHDAI) Workshop | GA | $98,792 |
| **Total (1 award)** | | | **$98,792** |

Source: GAO analysis of HHS information.

## Activity: Public Health Research

The purpose of this activity is to fund research projects through the ACA Prevention and Public Health Fund that investigate the effectiveness of public health services and systems in real world settings. The specific requirements for projects to be supported within this initiative are to (1) examine evidence-based practices related to prevention, with a particular focus on high-priority areas consistent with the National Prevention Strategy and Healthy People 2020, including comparisons of community-based public health interventions in terms of effectiveness and cost; (2) analyze the effective translation of interventions from academic settings to real world settings; and (3) identify effective strategies to organize, finance, or deliver public health services in real world community settings, including comparisons of state and local health department structures and systems in terms of effectiveness and cost.

- **Fiscal year 2010**: None

- **Fiscal year 2011**: $19.9 million (12 grants in three funding announcements totaling $11.5 million and 12 contracts totaling $8.4 million)

**Table 45: FY 2011 Grants, Public Health Research**

| Announcements (3) | Recipient | State | Award (dollars) |
|---|---|---|---|
| 1. Public Health Prevention Fund: Streamlined Surveillance for Ventilator-Associated Pneumonia: Reducing Burden and Demonstrating Preventability (RFA-CK11-001010PPHF11) | Harvard Pilgrim Health Care | MA | $1,544,184 |
| | **Total (1 award)** | | **$1,544,184** |
| **Purpose (award type)**: To evaluate the performance characteristics of streamlined ventilator associated pneumonia and evaluate the extent to which it can be prevented through adherence to process measures outlined in the HHS Action Plan. (Supplement) | | | |
| **Legislative Authority**: Section 307 of the Public Health Service Act as amended (42 U.S.C. 242l). | | | |
| **Eligibility**: Applicants selected as a Prevention Epicenter under FOA CK 11-001. | | | |
| 2. Preparedness and Emergency Response Research Centers: A Public Health Systems Approach (RFA-TP-08-001) | University of California, Berkeley | CA | $1,509,000 |
| | University of California, Los Angeles | CA | 1,197,000 |
| **Purpose (award type)**: To fund research for promoting and enhancing the preparedness and emergency response capabilities of the public health infrastructure at the federal, state, local, and tribal levels. (New) | University of Minnesota | MN | 1,147,000 |
| | University of North Carolina, Chapel Hill | NC | 1,147,000 |
| | **Total (4 awards)** | | **$5,000,000** |
| **Legislative Authority**: Section 319F(d)(7) of the Public Health Service Act, 42 U.S.C. 247d-6(d)(7). | | | |
| **Eligibility**: Accredited Schools of Public Health, as required by section 319F-2(d) of the Public Health Service Act. Only schools accredited by the Council on Education for Public Health are eligible | | | |
| 3. Preparedness and Emergency Response Learning Centers (CDC-RFA-TP10-100102CONT11) | University of South Florida | FL | $714,285 |
| | Johns Hopkins University | MD | 714,286 |
| **Purpose (award type)**: To address legislative requirements, as stated in section 319F(d) of the Public Health Service (PHS) Act (42 USC § 247d-6(d), as part of a plan to improve the nation's public health and medical preparedness and response capabilities for emergencies, whether deliberate, accidental, or natural. (New) | University of Albany, SUNY | NY | 714,286 |
| | Columbia University | NY | 714,286 |
| | University of Oklahoma | OK | 714,286 |
| | Texas A & M University | TX | 714,286 |
| **Legislative Authority**: Section 319F(d) of the Public Health Service (PHS) Act (42 USC § 247d-6(d)). | University of Washington | WA | 714,285 |
| | **Total (7 awards)** | | **$5,000,000** |
| **Eligibility**: Accredited Schools of Public Health that received their accreditation from the Council on Education for Public Health. | | | |

Source: GAO analysis of HHS information.

**Table 46: FY 2011 Contracts, Public Health Research**

| Recipient | Purpose | State | Award (dollars) |
|---|---|---|---|
| Healthy Housing Solutions Inc | Tobacco Control: Adoption, Health Impact and Cost of Smoke-Free Multi-Unit Housing Policies | GA | $2,210,000 |
| Research Service, Hines VA Hospital | Evaluating the impact of a treatment intervention to reduce Clostridium difficile transmission from asymptomatic C. difficile carriers in VA Community Living Centers | GA | 1,846,000 |
| The Johns Hopkins University | Center of Excellence for Measuring the Health and Social Impacts of Changes in State Alcohol Prices | GA | 1,636,598 |
| University of North Carolina at Chapel Hill | The Effectiveness of extending a "Consistent Care" program aimed to prevent prescription drug overdoses | NC | 745,000 |
| Washington State University | A randomized controlled trial of proactive reporting by prescription drug monitoring programs (PDMP) | WA | 550,587 |
| ABT Associates Inc. | A randomized controlled trial of proactive reporting by prescription drug monitoring programs (PDMP) | MD | 505,514 |
| Emergint Technologies, Inc. | Promoting DVT/PE prevention through monitoring practices and health outcomes | GA | 321,045 |
| Goodwill Industries of North Georgia | CDC Program Oversight & Implementation | GA | 250,000 |
| Lantana Consulting Group | HL7 Implementation Guidance Development and Maintenance | GA | 128,955 |
| Deloitte Consulting, LLP | CDC Program Oversight & Implementation | GA | 100,000 |
| Avaris Concepts, LLC | Logistical support of the s-VAP workgroup meeting | GA | 54,998 |
| Deloitte Consulting, LLP | CDC Program Oversight & Implementation | GA | 50,000 |
| **Total (12 awards)** | | | **$8,398,697** |

Source: GAO analysis of HHS information.

**Activity**: Community Guide/Community Preventive Services Task Force

The purpose of this activity is to help people choose programs and policies to improve health and prevent disease in communities using the Community Guide, a free resource. The activity's findings are used by partners at federal, state, and local levels within governments, health departments, worksites, community-based organizations, and elsewhere to guide and improve public health programs, policies, and research.

- **Fiscal year 2010**: $5.0 million (six grants in one funding announcement totaling $2.2 million and six contracts totaling $2.8 million)

- **Fiscal year 2011**: $6.0 million (six grants in one funding announcement totaling $1.3 million and seven contracts totaling $4.7 million)

**Table 47: FY 2010 Grants, Community Guide/Community Preventive Services Task Force**

| Announcement | Recipient | State | Award (dollars) |
|---|---|---|---|
| Affordable Care Act: Capacity Building Assistance to Strengthen Public Health Infrastructure and Performance (CDC-RFA-HM08-8050301SUPP10) | National Association of City/County Health Officials | DC | $500,000 |
| **Purpose (award type)**: To expand funding announcement CDC-RFA-HM08-805 by supporting the provision of capacity building assistance to state, tribal, local and territorial health departments that ensures successful adoption of best or promising practices to address key areas of public health infrastructure investments. (Supplement) | Association of State and Territorial Health Officials | VA | 500,000 |
| | National Network of Public Health Institutes | LA | 450,000 |
| | Public Health Foundation | DC | 350,000 |
| | National Association of Local Boards of Health | OH | 300,000 |
| | Association of Maternal and Child Health Programs | DC | 100,000 |
| **Legislative Authority**: Sections 301 and 317 of the Public Health Service Act (PHS Act), 42 USC, 241 and 247b as amended. Funding is appropriated under the Affordable Care Act (PL 111-148), Title IV, Section 4002 (Prevention and Public Health Fund). | **Total (6 awards)** | | **$2,200,000** |
| **Eligibility**: Limited to specific national, non-profit, public health professional organizations funded through the competitive funding announcement CDC-RFA-HM08-805. | | | |

Source: GAO analysis of HHS information.

**Table 48: FY 2010 Contracts, Community Guide/Community Preventive Services Task Force**

| Recipient | Purpose | State | Award (dollars) |
|---|---|---|---|
| Dept of Energy/Oak Ridge Ops | Collection, Review & Analysis of Data | GA | $1,300,000 |
| Westat | Community Guide Communication Technical Assistance and Support | MD | 1,054,685 |
| Deloitte Consulting, LLP | Business services support - Financial Management Office | GA | 180,000 |
| Chickasaw Advisory Services, LLC | Provide analytical epidemiology support | GA | 122,500 |
| Chickasaw Advisory Services, LLC | Provide analytical epidemiology support | GA | 122,500 |
| Deloitte Consulting, LLP | Business services support - Health Reform Implementation Office | GA | 20,000 |
| **Total (6 awards)** | | | **$2,799,685** |

Source: GAO analysis of HHS information.

**Table 49: FY 2011 Grants, Community Guide/Community Preventive Services Task Force**

| Announcement | Recipient | State | Award (dollars) |
|---|---|---|---|
| Non-Competitive 12-month Cost Extension Supplement for CDC-RFA-HM08-8050301SUPP10: Affordable Care Act (ACA): Capacity Building Assistance to Strengthen Public Health Infrastructure and Performance (CDC-RFA-HM08-8050401PPHF11) | Association of State and Territorial Health Officials | VA | $305,682 |
| | Public Health Foundation | DC | 296,329 |
| | National Association of City/County Health Officials | DC | 266,821 |
| | National Network of Public Health Institutes | LA | 249,582 |
| **Purpose (award type)**: To expand funding announcement CDC-RFA-HM08-805 by supporting the provision of capacity building assistance to state, tribal, local and territorial health departments that ensures performance improvement and successful adoption of best or promising practices to address key areas of public health infrastructure investments. (Supplement) | National Association of Local Boards of Health | OH | 165,449 |
| | Association of Maternal and Child Health Programs | DC | 61,137 |
| | **Total (6 awards)** | | **$1,345,000** |
| **Legislative Authority**: Sections 301 and 317 of the Public Health Service Act (PHS Act), 42 USC, 241 and 247b as amended. Funding is appropriated under the Affordable Care Act (PL 111-148), Title IV, Section 4002 (Prevention and Public Health Fund) | | | |
| **Eligibility**: Eligibility is limited to specific national, non-profit, public health professional organizations funded through the funding announcement CDC-RFA-HM08-8030301SUPP10. | | | |

Source: GAO analysis of HHS information.

**Table 50: FY 2011 Contracts, Community Guide/Community Preventive Services Task Force**

| Recipient | Purpose | State | Award (dollars) |
|---|---|---|---|
| Cloudburst Consulting Group, INC. | Programmatic Management/ Intramural HR | GA | $1,499,286 |
| Department of Energy | ORISE Fellows | GA | 1,300,000 |
| University of Manchester | Low Complexity Community Guide Reviews | GA | 886,350 |
| Westat, Inc. | Communications Support Contract | GA | 629,976 |
| Deloitte Consulting, LLP | CDC Program Oversight & Implementation | GA | 245,000 |
| Chickasaw Advisory Services, LLC | Health Scientist | GA | 99,809 |
| Deloitte Consulting, LLP | CDC Program Oversight & Implementation | GA | 35,000 |
| **Total (7 awards)** | | | **$4,695,421** |

Source: GAO analysis of HHS information.

**Activity**: Healthcare-Associated Infections (HAI)

The purpose of this activity is to expand state prevention activities through funding to health departments that have already demonstrated successes and capacity to implement HAI prevention programs and to build upon advances made through Recovery Act investments. This program is designed to accelerate electronic reporting to detect HAIs at the state level by decreasing data entry burden. Electronic reporting will increase validation of data and the ability of states and healthcare facilities to measure the impact of prevention efforts.

- **Fiscal year 2010**: None

- **Fiscal year 2011**: $11.4 million (54 grants in two funding announcements totaling $9.4 million and four contracts totaling $2.0 million)

Table 51: FY 2011 Grants, Healthcare-Associated Infections

| Announcements (2) | Recipient | State | Award (dollars) |
|---|---|---|---|
| 1. Patient Protection and Affordable Care Act Epidemiology and Laboratory Capacity for Infectious Diseases Building and Strengthening Epidemiology, Laboratory and Health Information Systems Capacity in State and Local Health Departments (CDC-RFA-CI10-101202PPHF11) | Michigan State Dept of Community Health | MI | $782,173 |
| | Illinois State Dept of Public Health | IL | 779,616 |
| | California Department of Public Health | CA | 771,473 |
| | Tennessee State Department of Health | TN | 768,006 |
| | New York State Dept of Health | NY | 621,473 |
| **Purpose (award type)**: To enhance public health programs that focus on improving health and helping restrain the rate of growth of health care costs through building epidemiology, laboratory, and health information systems capacity in state and local public health departments. (Continuation) | Massachusetts State Dept of Pub Health | MA | 521,473 |
| | Oregon State Public Health Division | OR | 426,523 |
| | Florida State Department of Health | FL | 421,472 |
| | Colorado State Dept/Pub Hlth & Environmt | CO | 363,303 |
| | Arizona State Department of Hlth Srvcs | AZ | 316,078 |
| **Legislative Authority**: Public Health Service Act Sections 301(a) [42 U.S.C. 241(a)] and 317(k) (2) [42 U.S.C. 247b (k) (2)], as amended and the Patient Protection and Affordable Care Act (PL 111-148), Title IV, Sections 4002 and 4304 (Prevention and Public Health Fund). | Nevada State Dept of Hlth/Human Svcs | NV | 296,516 |
| | KY Cabinet for Health and Family Services | KY | 274,784 |
| | Minnesota State Dept of Health | MN | 71,474 |
| | Mississippi State Department of Health | MS | 71,473 |
| | Montana State Dept/Pub Hlth & Human Srvs | MT | 71,473 |
| **Eligibility**: Limited to 58 state and local public health departments or their established bona fide agents that were 2010 grantees of Epidemiology and Laboratory Capacity for Infectious Diseases CI10-1012 funding announcement. | NH State Dept of Health and Human Sers | NH | 71,473 |
| | New Jersey State Dept/Health/Senior Srvs | NJ | 71,473 |
| | New Mexico State Department of Health | NM | 71,473 |
| | Ohio State Department of Health | OH | 71,473 |
| | Pennsylvania State Dept of Health | PA | 71,473 |
| | Virginia State Dept of Health | VA | 71,473 |
| | Alabama State Dept of Public Health | AL | 71,472 |
| | Alaska State Department of Hlth-Soc Svcs | AK | 71,472 |
| | Georgia Department of Community Health | GA | 71,472 |
| | Indiana State Department of Health | IN | 71,472 |
| | Iowa State Dept of Public Health | IA | 71,472 |
| | Kansas State Dept of Hlth and Environmnt | KS | 71,472 |
| | Maine State Dept/Health/Human Servs | ME | 71,472 |
| | NC State Dept/Hlth & Human Services | NC | 71,472 |
| | Oklahoma State Department of Health | OK | 71,472 |
| | Wisconsin Department of Health Services | WI | 71,472 |
| | Arkansas State Dept of Health | AR | 71,471 |
| | South Carolina State Dept of Hlth/Env | SC | 71,252 |
| | Hawaii State Department of Health | HI | 70,992 |
| | Connecticut State Dept of Public Health | CT | 69,980 |

| Announcements (2) | Recipient | State | Award (dollars) |
|---|---|---|---|
| | Vermont Department of Health | VT | 67,236 |
| | Maryland State Dept of Hlth/Mtl Hygiene | MD | 66,852 |
| | Delaware State Dept of Hlth & Soc Srvs | DE | 66,760 |
| | Nebraska St Dept of Health & Human Servs | NE | 66,300 |
| | Puerto Rico Department of Health | PR | 66,154 |
| | Washington State Department of Health | WA | 66,153 |
| | Rhode Island State Dept of Health | RI | 66,147 |
| | Missouri State Dept/ Health & Senior Srv | MO | 66,121 |
| | South Dakota State Dept of Health | SD | 63,945 |
| | DC Department of Health | DC | 63,342 |
| | West Virginia State Dept Hlth/Human Rscs | WV | 62,760 |
| | Idaho State Dept of Health And Welfare | ID | 58,617 |
| | Utah State Department of Health | UT | 55,647 |
| | North Dakota State Department of Health | ND | 48,611 |
| | Louisiana State Dept of Hlth & Hospitals | LA | 47,553 |
| | Wyoming State Department of Health | WY | 23,239 |
| | **Total (51 awards)** | | **$8,939,999**[a] |
| 2. Competitive Program Expansion Supplement for CDC-RFA-HM08-805: Strengthen and Improve the Nation's Capacity through National, Non-profit, Professional Public Health Organizations to Increase Health Protection and Health Equity (CDC-RFA-HM08-8050402PHFF11) | Council of State and Territorial Epidemiologists | GA | $290,000 |
| | National Association of City/County Health Officials | DC | 100,000 |
| | Association of State and Territorial Health Officials | VA | 100,000 |
| | **Total (3 awards)** | | **$490,000** |

**Purpose (award type)**: Support the provision of capacity building assistance to state, tribal, local and territorial health departments that ensures performance improvement and successful adoption of best or promising practices to address key areas of public health infrastructure investments. (Supplement)

**Legislative Authority**: Sections 301 and 317 of the Public Health Service Act (PHS Act), 42 USC, 241 and 247b as amended. Funding is appropriated under the Affordable Care Act (PL 111-148), Title IV, Section 4002 (Prevention and Public Health Fund).

**Eligibility**: Limited to specific national, non-profit, public health professional organizations funded through the competitive funding opportunity announcement CDC-RFA-HM08-805.

Source: GAO analysis of HHS information.

[a]Column does not total due to rounding.

Table 52: FY 2011 Contracts, Healthcare-Associated Infections

| Recipient | Purpose | State | Award (dollars) |
|---|---|---|---|
| Science Applications International Corporation (SAIC) | National Healthcare Safety Network (NHSN) development and infrastructure requirements for surveillance of HAIs | VA | $1,065,693 |
| Four Seasons Environmental, Inc. | CDC Program Oversight & Implementation | GA | 470,000 |
| Lantana Consulting Group | HL7 Implementation Guidance Development and Maintenance | GA | 434,307 |
| Avaris Concepts, LLC | DHQP's State-based Training Activity & Resource Support (STARS) Training and Resource Initiative | GA | 50,000 |
| Total (4 awards) | | | $2,020,000 |

Source: GAO analysis of HHS information.

### Activity: Prevention Research Centers

The purpose of this activity is to help alter the individual behaviors and community environmental factors that put people at risk for the leading causes of death and disability—chronic diseases, such as cancer, heart disease, and diabetes. Centers may also address risks for injury, infectious disease, mental health, global health, and the health effects of impairments such as deafness. The activity is designed to bridge gaps between research findings and the translation of those findings into public health practice and policy.

- **Fiscal year 2010:** None

- **Fiscal year 2011**: $10.0 million (15 grants in one funding announcement)

**Table 53: FY 2011 Grants, Prevention Research Centers**

| Announcement | Recipient | State | Award (dollars) |
|---|---|---|---|
| Health Promotion and Disease Prevention Research Centers (RFA-DP09-00103SUPP11) | University of Arizona | AZ | $1,015,000 |
| | San Diego State University with (UCSD) | CA | 965,000 |
| **Purpose (award type)**: To support a network of Health Promotion and Disease Prevention Research Centers that: (1) focus on the major causes of disease and disability, with an emphasis on underserved and minority populations; (2) improve public health practice through a community-based participatory research process; and (3) design, test, disseminate, or translate effective public health programs at the state and community levels. Funded centers will also function as a part of a networked environment to support and advance health promotion and disease prevention research and serve as a national resource for developing and applying effective public health programs at the state or community level. (New) | Morehouse School of Medicine | GA | 894,500 |
| | NYU Medical Center | NY | 785,999 |
| | University of Rochester | NY | 744,501 |
| | West Virginia University Research Corporation | WV | 690,000 |
| | Yale University | CT | 615,000 |
| | University of South Florida | FL | 615,000 |
| | Johns Hopkins University | MD | 615,000 |
| | Boston University | MA | 615,000 |
| | University of New Mexico | NM | 615,000 |
| | Case Western Reserve University | OH | 615,000 |
| **Legislative Authority**: Section 1706 of the Public Health Service Act (PHS Act), 42 U.S.C. 300u-5, as amended. | Oregon Health and Science University | OR | 615,000 |
| | University of Maryland | MD | 300,000 |
| **Eligibility**: Accredited schools of public health and accredited schools of osteopathy and accredited schools of medicine that offer an accredited Preventive Medicine Residency program. Osteopathy and medicine schools in the process of obtaining accreditation for a Preventive Medicine Residency program are also eligible. | Dartmouth College | NH | 300,000 |
| | **Total (15 awards)** | | **$10,000,000** |

Source: GAO analysis of HHS information.

## Activity: Workplace Wellness

The purpose of this activity is to engage and recruit through a national organization, groups of 10-15 employers and lead them through the process of building a core workplace health program.

- **Fiscal year 2010**: None

- **Fiscal year 2011**: $9.2 million (six contracts)

**Table 54: FY 2011 Contracts, Workplace Wellness**

| Recipient | Purpose | State | Award (dollars) |
|---|---|---|---|
| Viridian Health Management | Worksite Wellness Program Contract | GA | $7,769,250 |
| Research Triangle Institute | Program Evaluation | GA | 537,824 |
| Carter Consulting, Inc. | Management Consultation and Technical Assistance Services | GA | 360,501 |
| Deloitte Consulting, LLP | CDC Program Oversight & Implementation | GA | 350,000 |
| Dell Services Federal Government, Inc. | IT Support | GA | 100,000 |
| Four Seasons Environmental, Inc. | CDC Program Oversight & Implementation | GA | 50,000 |
| **Total (6 awards)** | | | **$9,167,575** |

Source: GAO analysis of HHS information.

## Activity: National Youth Fitness Survey

The purpose of this activity is to gather data on physical activity and fitness in children and teens through the National Youth Fitness Survey. The survey is conducted by the National Center for Health Statistics, part of the Centers for Disease Control and Prevention.

- **Fiscal year 2010**: None

- **Fiscal year 2011**: $5.9 million (four contracts)

**Table 55: FY 2011 Contracts, National Youth Fitness Survey**

| Recipient | Purpose | State | Award (dollars) |
|---|---|---|---|
| Westat | National Youth Fitness Survey Activities | MD | $5,305,291 |
| Westat | Trailer refurbishment | MD | 354,709 |
| Four Seasons Environmental | CDC Program Oversight & Implementation | GA | 210,000 |
| Deloitte Consulting | CDC Program Oversight & Implementation | GA | 30,000 |
| **Total (4 awards)** | | | **$5,900,000** |

Source: GAO analysis of HHS information.

## Activity: ARRA: Evaluation

The purpose of this activity is to support the Behavioral Risk Factor
Surveillance System (BRFSS) in tracking health conditions and risk
behaviors in the United States.

- **Fiscal year 2010**: $4.0 million (nine grants in one funding
  announcement totaling $3.6 million and five contracts totaling
  $0.4 million)

- **Fiscal year 2011**: None

**Table 56: FY 2010 Grants, ARRA: Evaluation**

| Announcement | Recipient | State | Award (dollars) |
|---|---|---|---|
| Patient Protection and Affordable Care Act (Affordable Care Act) State Competitive Supplemental Funding for Behavioral Risk Factor Surveillance System (CDC-RFA-DP09-90103-SUPP10) | Arkansas State Dept of Health | AR | $892,025 |
| | North Carolina State Dept/Hlth & Human Services | NC | 772,104 |
| | Alabama State Dept of Public Health | AL | 749,995 |
| | Pinellas County Health Dept | FL | 500,000 |
| **Purpose (award type):** To provide State Health Departments with resources to maintain previous projections in sample size, enhance and expand the utility of Behavioral Risk Factor Surveillance System, and support ongoing state-based public health surveillance infrastructure. (Supplement) | Florida State Department of Health | FL | 326,905 |
| | Georgia Department of Community Health | GA | 109,533 |
| | Illinois State Dept of Public Health | IL | 99,845 |
| | Texas State Dept of Health Services | TX | 75,148 |
| **Legislative Authority:** Sections 301, 307, 310, and 311 of the Public Health Service Act, as amended, and the Comprehensive Smoking Education Act of 1984, Comprehensive Smokeless Tobacco Health Education Act of 1986, and Patient Protection and Affordable Care Act (Affordable Care Act). | Dekalb County Board of Public Health | GA | 61,000 |
| | **Total (9 awards)** | | **$3,586,555** |
| **Eligibility:** All 50 states, the District of Columbia, Puerto Rico and U.S. Virgin Islands. Eligibility for the evaluation of Communities Putting Prevention to Work component is limited to state health departments in which a Communities Putting Prevention to Work grantee resides within the state health agency jurisdiction boundary. | | | |

Source: GAO analysis of HHS information.

**Table 57: FY 2010 Contracts, ARRA: Evaluation**

| Recipient | Purpose | State | Award (dollars) |
|---|---|---|---|
| Denali Corporation DBA Denali Technologies | BRFSS data evaluation | GA | $120,132 |
| WESTAT | Fund the sampling and weighting of BRFSS data once it has been collected by ARRA/CPPW communities through this point in time surveys. | GA | 106,171 |
| Deloitte Consulting, LLP | Business services support - Financial Management Office | GA | 70,296 |
| Northrop Grumman | Support all aspects of full lifecycle application systems development and maintenance on a variety of platforms including mainframe, client server, and web; architecture and infrastructure design to support enterprise application software services including hardware/software/network design and implementation; database design, application development and support; data management and security controls; quality assurance, test and control functions; and technical communication, consultation and information support. | GA | 59,209 |
| Deloitte Consulting, LLP | Business services support - Health Reform Implementation Office | GA | 10,000 |
| **Total (5 awards)** | | | **$365,808** |

Source: GAO analysis of HHS information.

## Activity: ARRA: Media

The purpose of this activity is to provide enhanced media buying/placement support to the National Prevention Media Initiative to increase exposure of audiences to campaign messages in communities that received Communities Putting Prevention to Work awards. The goal of this activity is to achieve maximum additional exposure of existing/in-development creative campaign materials.

- **Fiscal year 2010**: $3.9 million (three contracts)

- **Fiscal year 2011**: None

**Table 58: FY 2010 Contracts, ARRA: Media**

| Recipient | Purpose | State | Award (dollars) |
|---|---|---|---|
| CAMPBELL-EWALD COMPANY | Advertising and marketing services for planning and execution of paid-media strategies in support of the National Prevention Media Initiative. | GA | $3,730,000 |
| Department of Health and Human Services | Provide publication development and management, Web development and maintenance, and other presentation and communication support | MO | 110,000 |
| Deloitte Consulting, LLP | Business services support - Health Reform Implementation Office | GA | 10,000 |
| **Total (3 awards)** | | | **$3,850,000** |

Source: GAO analysis of HHS information.

## Activity: Education and Outreach Campaign Regarding Preventive Benefits

The purpose of this activity is to support the Pharmacy Outreach Project to increase pharmacists' capacity and interest in providing over-the-counter advice to patients with high blood pressure, especially encouraging medication adherence and the use of available preventive clinical services.

- **Fiscal year 2010**: None

- **Fiscal year 2011**: $1.8 million (four contracts)

**Table 59: FY 2011 Contracts, Education and Outreach Campaign Regarding Preventive Benefits**

| Recipient | Purpose | State | Award (dollars) |
|---|---|---|---|
| Ogilvy Public Relations Worldwide Inc. | Communications Support for Pharmacists Partnership and Cardiovascular Disease Prevention Activities | GA | $1,696,945 |
| Four Seasons Environmental, Inc. | CDC Program Oversight & Implementation | GA | 70,000 |
| Northrup Grumman Systems Corporation | CDC Program Oversight & Implementation | GA | 15,000 |
| Deloitte Consulting, LLP | CDC Program Oversight & Implementation | GA | 10,000 |
| **Total (4 awards)** | | | **$1,791,945** |

Source: GAO analysis of HHS information.

## Activity: National Prevention Strategy

The purpose of this activity is to guide our nation in the most effective and achievable way to improve health and well being; the National Prevention Strategy prioritizes prevention by integrating recommendations and actions across multiple settings to improve health and save lives.

- **Fiscal year 2010**: $0.01 million (one contract)

- **Fiscal year 2011**: $0.7 million (four contracts)

**Table 60: FY 2010 Contract, National Prevention Strategy**

| Recipient | Purpose | State | Award (dollars) |
|---|---|---|---|
| Northrop Grumman | Support all aspects of full lifecycle application systems development and maintenance on a variety of platforms including mainframe, client server, and web; architecture and infrastructure design to support enterprise application software services including hardware/software/network design and implementation; database design, application development and support; data management and security controls; quality assurance, test and control functions; and technical communication, consultation and information support. | GA | $14,500 |
| **Total (1 award)** | | | **$14,500** |

Source: GAO analysis of HHS information.

**Table 61: FY 2011 Contracts, National Prevention Strategy**

| Recipient | Purpose | State | Award (dollars) |
|---|---|---|---|
| Deloitte Consulting, LLP | Strategic & Tactical Planning, Workforce Development and other Related Transformation Initiatives | GA | $529,525 |
| Department of Energy | Research Participation Program | GA | 98,000 |
| Deloitte Consulting, LLP | CDC Program Oversight & Implementation | GA | 35,000 |
| Goodwill Industries of North GA | CDC Program Oversight & Implementation | GA | 5,000 |
| **Total (4 awards)** | | | **$667,525** |

Source: GAO analysis of HHS information.

## Activity: Promoting Obesity Prevention in Early Childhood Programs

The purpose of this activity is to encourage child care providers across the nation to adopt healthier policies and practices around physical activity and nutrition, including limiting screen time and supporting breastfeeding.

- **Fiscal year 2010**: None

- **Fiscal year 2011**: $0.7 million (seven contracts)

**Table 62: FY 2011 Contracts, Promoting Obesity Prevention in Early Childhood Programs**

| Recipient | Purpose | State | Award (dollars) |
|---|---|---|---|
| National Institutes of Health | CDC support for NCCOR coordinating and collaborating projects | GA | $200,000 |
| McKing Consulting Corporation | Management Consultation and Technical Assistance | GA | 194,969 |
| The Regents of the University of Colorado | Development of a comprehensive state policy evaluation for nutrition, physical activity and obesity (University of Colorado, Denver) | CO | 150,000 |
| Department of Energy | Collaborative efforts to prevent obesity in early childhood | GA | 93,031 |
| FHI Development 360 LLC | ORISE: Nutrition and Physical Activity Research | GA | 80,001 |
| Deloitte Consulting, LLP | CDC Program Oversight & Implementation | GA | 28,000 |
| Four Seasons Environmental, Inc. | CDC Program Oversight & Implementation | GA | 2,000 |
| **Total (7 awards)** | | | **$748,001** |

Source: GAO analysis of HHS information.

# Appendix III: Health Resources and Services Administration—Prevention and Public Health Fund Awards by Activity

This appendix presents information on awards made by the Health Resources and Services Administration (HRSA) for Prevention and Public Health Fund (PPHF) activities with funds allocated and transferred from the PPHF for fiscal years (FY) 2010 and 2011. For each HRSA activity that received PPHF funding, tables 63 through 70 summarize information on awards made with those funds through grants and contracts for each fiscal year.[1] Award information was provided by HHS's Assistant Secretary for Financial Resources, HRSA, or reported in the funding opportunity announcements (FOA) HHS identified as being associated with the activity and awards.

The information presented in this appendix, including the purpose of the PPHF-funded activity, was obtained from HHS. Due to the large number of awards, we did not edit the award recipient information to correct typographical or grammatical errors, or clarify the information provided. In general, we reprinted the abbreviations and acronyms provided by HHS and the legislative authority cited in the FOA or otherwise provided by HHS. We did not independently verify the legislative authority. Totals in this appendix (reported obligations) may not match—for example, they may be less than—the amounts in table 2 (reported allocations). According to HHS officials, to carry out an activity, an agency may incur administrative expenses, including internal costs associated with managing and overseeing grants and contracts, not reflected in award amounts. Further, to the extent that an appropriation has not identified a particular amount for a specific activity, an agency may reallocate unobligated funds from that activity to another during the course of a fiscal year.

**Activity**: Primary Care Training and Enhancement

The purpose of this activity is to support and develop primary care physician and physician assistant programs. The program deploys its resources to strengthen medical education for physician and physician assistants to improve the quantity, quality, distribution, and diversity of the primary care workforce.

---

[1]The tables present information on cooperative agreements with grants, and include information on interagency agreements with contracts.

- **Fiscal year 2010**: $197.5 million (110 grants in two funding announcements)

- **Fiscal year 2011**: None

**Table 63: FY 2010 Grants, Primary Care Training and Enhancement**

| Announcements (2) | Recipient[a] | State | Award (dollars) |
|---|---|---|---|
| 1. Primary Care Residency Expansion Program (HRSA-10-277) | Children's Hospital & Research Center at Oakland | CA | $3,840,000 |
| | Children's National Medical Center | DC | 3,840,000 |
| **Purpose (award type)**: To increase the number of primary care physicians by expanding enrollment in accredited primary care residency programs, including family medicine, general internal, and general pediatric medicine. The program funds resident support of $80,000 per resident per year for a total of three years per resident. (New) | Boston Medical Center | MA | 3,840,000 |
| | Baystate Medical Center | MA | 3,840,000 |
| | The Ohio State University | OH | 3,840,000 |
| | Johns Hopkins University | MD | 3,839,998 |
| | University of North Carolina At Chapel Hill | NC | 3,715,684 |
| | Spectrum Health Hospitals | MI | 3,490,659 |
| **Legislative Authority**: Section 747 of the Public Health Service Act (42 U.S.C. 293k), as amended by section 5301 of the Patient Protection and Affordable Care Act (Pub. L. 111-148), and section 4002 of the Patient Protection and Affordable Care Act (Publ. L. 111-148). | Danbury Hospital | CT | 3,360,000 |
| | Louisiana State University Health Science Center | LA | 3,120,000 |
| | Regents of University of California | CA | 2,880,000 |
| | Baystate Medical Center | MA | 2,880,000 |
| | Bronx-Lebanon Hosp Ctr | NY | 2,880,000 |
| | Bronx-Lebanon Hosp Ctr | NY | 2,880,000 |
| **Eligibility**: Public or nonprofit private hospitals, schools of medicine or osteopathic medicine, or a public or private nonprofit entity which the Secretary has determined is capable of carrying out such grants. An applicant must be accredited as a residency training program in family medicine, general internal medicine, and/or general pediatrics by the Accreditation Council for Graduate Medical Education (ACGME) or by the American Osteopathic Association (AOA). | Kingsbrook Jewish Medical Center | NY | 2,880,000 |
| | Richmond Medical Center | NY | 2,880,000 |
| | The Reading Hospital And Medical Center | PA | 2,880,000 |
| | Meharry Medical College | TN | 2,880,000 |
| | Mount Auburn Hospital | MA | 2,879,998 |
| | Variety Children's Hospital dba Miami Children's Hospital | FL | 2,861,568 |
| | University of Pennsylvania | PA | 2,777,757 |
| | Tulane University, School of Medicine | LA | 2,472,964 |
| | Texas Tech University Health Sciences Center | TX | 1,920,001 |
| | Regents of the University of California | CA | 1,920,000 |
| | Catholic Healthcare West/St. Mary Medical Center | CA | 1,920,000 |
| | The Regents of the University of California, Los Angeles | CA | 1,920,000 |
| | Regents of the University of California | CA | 1,920,000 |
| | The Regents of the University of California, San Francisco | CA | 1,920,000 |
| | The Regents of the University of California, San Francisco | CA | 1,920,000 |

| Announcements (2) | Recipient[a] | State | Award (dollars) |
|---|---|---|---|
| | Regents of the University of Colorado | CO | 1,920,000 |
| | University of Colorado Denver | CO | 1,920,000 |
| | University of Florida | FL | 1,920,000 |
| | The University of Illinois At Chicago | IL | 1,920,000 |
| | Central Iowa Hospital Corporation | IA | 1,920,000 |
| | Curators, University of Missouri on behalf of UMKC | MO | 1,920,000 |
| | Curators, University of Missouri On Behalf of UMKC | MO | 1,920,000 |
| | Cooper Health System D/B/A Cooper University Hospital | NJ | 1,920,000 |
| | Cooper Health System D/B/A Cooper University Hospital | NJ | 1,920,000 |
| | Newark Beth Israel Medical Center | NJ | 1,920,000 |
| | Newark Beth Israel Medical Center | NJ | 1,920,000 |
| | University of Medicine and Dentistry of New Jersey | NJ | 1,920,000 |
| | St. Elizabeth Medical Center | NY | 1,920,000 |
| | Crozer-Chester Medical Center | PA | 1,920,000 |
| | Albert Einstein Healthcare Network | PA | 1,920,000 |
| | Children's Hospital of Pittsburgh of the UPMC Health System | PA | 1,920,000 |
| | Medical University of South Carolina | SC | 1,920,000 |
| | The University of Texas Southwestern Medical Center At Dallas | TX | 1,920,000 |
| | Baylor College of Medicine | TX | 1,920,000 |
| | Carilion Medical Center | VA | 1,920,000 |
| | Community Health of Central Washington | WA | 1,920,000 |
| | Marshfield Clinic Research Foundation | WI | 1,920,000 |
| | Marshfield Clinic Research Foundation | WI | 1,920,000 |
| | Hennepin Healthcare System, Inc/Hennepin County Medical Center | MN | 1,918,827 |
| | Sisters of Charity Hospital | NY | 1,912,499 |
| | Variety Children's Hospital Doing dba Miami Children's Hospital | FL | 1,907,712 |
| | Freeman Oak Hill Health System | MO | 1,907,712 |
| | University of Connecticut Health Center | CT | 1,890,723 |
| | University of Rochester | NY | 1,887,125 |
| | Cincinnati Children's Hospital Medical Center | OH | 1,872,024 |
| | Board of Trustees of Southern Illinois University | IL | 1,869,763 |
| | New Hanover Regional Medical Center | NC | 1,795,571 |
| | Virginia Commonwealth University | VA | 1,585,520 |
| | University of Arkansas for Medical Sciences | AR | 1,520,001 |

| Announcements (2) | Recipient[a] | State | Award (dollars) |
|---|---|---|---|
| | University of Arkansas for Medical Sciences-Cancer Research Center | AR | 1,520,001 |
| | Montefiore Medical Center | NY | 1,490,111 |
| | Yellowstone City & County Health Department/Riverstone Health | MT | 960,003 |
| | The Family Medicine Residency of Idaho, Inc. | ID | 960,000 |
| | The Family Medicine Residency of Idaho, Inc. | ID | 960,000 |
| | Idaho State University | ID | 960,000 |
| | Swedish Covenant Hospital | IL | 960,000 |
| | Community Hospitals Foundation | IN | 960,000 |
| | Univ. of Mass. Medical School | MA | 960,000 |
| | The Regents of the University of Michigan | MI | 960,000 |
| | Board of Regents, University of Nevada, Reno | NV | 960,000 |
| | UMDNJ – Robert Wood Johnson Medical School | NJ | 960,000 |
| | UPMC Presbyterian Shadyside | PA | 960,000 |
| | Baylor Research Institute | TX | 960,000 |
| | Texas Tech Univ Health Sciences Center | TX | 960,000 |
| | Providence St Peter Hospital | WA | 960,000 |
| | Group Health Cooperative | WA | 960,000 |
| | University of Arkansas | AR | 759,999 |
| | University of Arkansas for Medical Sciences-Cancer Research Center | AR | 759,999 |
| | **Total (82 awards)** | | **$167,356,219** |
| 2. Expansion of Physician Assistant Training (EPAT) Program (HRSA-10-278)<br><br>**Purpose (award type)**: To increase student enrollment in primary care Physician Assistant programs and graduates planning to practice primary care specialties. The program funds physician assistant student stipends, educational expenses, reasonable living expenses and indirect costs for a total of $22,000 per student, for a maximum of two years per student, plus indirect costs. (New) | Riverside Community College District/Moreno Valley Campus | CA | $2,117,808 |
| | The Research Foundation of SUNY | NY | 2,046,528 |
| | University of Texas-Pan American | TX | 1,980,000 |
| | University of Washington | WA | 1,980,000 |
| | Lincoln Memorial University | TN | 1,900,800 |
| | Grand Valley State University | MI | 1,791,720 |
| | Duke University Medical Center | NC | 1,320,000 |
| | Samuel Merritt College | CA | 1,232,000 |

| Announcements (2) | Recipient[a] | State | Award (dollars) |
|---|---|---|---|
| **Legislative Authority**: Section 747 of the Public Health Service Act (42 U.S.C. 293k), as amended by section 5301 of the Patient Protection and Affordable Care Act (Pub. L. 111-148), and section 4002 of the Patient Protection and Affordable Care Act (Pub. L. 111-148). | Methodist University, Inc. | NC | 1,188,000 |
| | Shenandoah University | VA | 1,069,200 |
| | LeMoyne College | NY | 1,056,000 |
| | The University of Toledo Health Science Campus | OH | 1,009,880 |
| | University of New England | ME | 990,000 |
| **Eligibility**: Public or private academically affiliated physician assistant training programs that have as their objective the education of individuals who, upon completion of their studies in the program, will be qualified to provide primary care medical services with the supervision of a physician. | King's College | PA | 990,000 |
| | University of Nebraska Medical Center | NE | 924,000 |
| | Chatham University | PA | 880,000 |
| | University of Colorado Denver | CO | 855,360 |
| | New York Institute of Technology | NY | 855,360 |
| | Union College | NE | 792,000 |
| | University of Southern California | CA | 704,000 |
| | Desales University | PA | 704,000 |
| | Marywood University | PA | 704,000 |
| | University of Utah | UT | 704,000 |
| | Pace University | NY | 660,000 |
| | Miami Dade College Medical Center Campus | FL | 641,520 |
| | The Univ. of Oklahoma Health Sciences Center | OK | 418,171 |
| | State of Colorado for Red Rocks Community College | CO | 399,495 |
| | University of New Mexico Health Sciences Center | NM | 204,239 |
| | **Total (28 awards)** | | **$30,118,081** |

Source: GAO analysis of HHS information.

[a]According to HRSA officials, applicants could submit applications for each accredited family medicine, general internal medicine, or general pediatric residency program in primary care provided by the institution, and could receive multiple awards.

## Activity: Public Health Workforce Development

The purpose of this activity is to support the training of public health workers. Public health workers protect and improve the health of communities through education, disease prevention and health promotion, and monitoring, diagnosis, research, and provision of services to address community health problems.

- **Fiscal year 2010**: $14.8 million (24 grants in one funding announcement)

- **Fiscal year 2011**: $20.0 million (32 grants in one funding announcement)

## Table 64: FY 2010 Grants, Public Health Workforce Development

| Announcement | Recipient | State | Award (dollars) |
|---|---|---|---|
| Public Health Training Centers Program (HRSA-10-270) | Regents of the University of California, Los Angeles | CA | $650,000 |
| | University of South Florida | FL | 650,000 |
| **Purpose (award type):** To improve the nation's public health system by strengthening the | Emory University | GA | 650,000 |
| technical, scientific, managerial, and leadership competence of the current and future public | The Regents of the Univ of Michigan | MI | 650,000 |
| health workforce. A public health training center | University of Puerto Rico Medical Sciences Campus | PR | 650,000 |
| plans, develops, operates, and evaluates projects that are in furtherance of the goals | University of South Carolina | SC | 650,000 |
| established by the Secretary in the areas of | East Tennessee State Univ | TN | 650,000 |
| preventive medicine, health promotion and | University of Washington | WA | 650,000 |
| disease prevention, or improving access to and quality of health services in medically | Univ of Pittsburgh | PA | 649,994 |
| underserved communities. (New) | Trustees of Boston University, BUMC | MA | 649,977 |
| **Legislative Authority**: Section 765 of the | The Research Foundation of SUNY | NY | 649,921 |
| Public Health Service Act (42 U.S.C. 295), as amended by section 5206 of the Patient | The Regents of the University of California | CA | 649,819 |
| Protection and Affordable Care Act | The Univ of Texas Health Science Center At Houston | TX | 649,801 |
| (Pub. L. 111-148), and section 766 of the Public Health Service Act (42 U.S.C. 295a), and | The University of Oklahoma Health Sciences Center | OK | 649,750 |
| section 4002 of the Patient Protection and | University of Colorado Denver | CO | 649,497 |
| Affordable Care Act (Publ. L. 111-148). | UMDNJ-School of Public Health | NJ | 647,654 |
| **Eligibility**: A Council on Education for Public | Arizona Board of Regents | AZ | 647,637 |
| Health (CEPH) accredited school of public health or another public or nonprofit private | University of Kentucky Research Foundation | KY | 647,307 |
| institution accredited for the provision of | Univ of North Carolina at Chapel Hill | NC | 643,004 |
| graduate or specialized training in public health. | The University of Georgia | GA | 630,032 |
| | Board of Regents of the University of Wisconsin System | WI | 628,480 |
| | Trustees of Dartmouth College | NH | 618,734 |
| | Eastern Virginia Medical School | VA | 488,360 |
| | Indiana University | IN | 129,267 |
| | **Total (24 awards)** | | **$14,829,234** |

Source: GAO analysis of HHS information.

**Table 65: FY 2011 Grants, Public Health Workforce Development**

| Announcement | Recipient | State | Award (dollars) |
|---|---|---|---|
| Public Health Training Centers Program (HRSA-11-142)<br><br>**Purpose (award type)**: To improve the nation's public health system by strengthening the technical, scientific, managerial, and leadership competence of the current and future public health workforce. A public health training center plans, develops, operates, and evaluates projects that are in furtherance of the goals established by the Secretary in the areas of preventive medicine, health promotion and disease prevention, or improving access to and quality of health services in medically underserved communities. (New and Continuation)<br><br>**Legislative Authority**: Section 765 of the Public Health Service Act (42 U.S.C. 295), as amended by section 5206 of the Patient Protection and Affordable Care Act (Pub. L. 111-148), and section 766 of the Public Health Service Act (42 U.S.C. 295a), and section 4002 of the Patient Protection and Affordable Care Act (Pub. L. 111-148).<br><br>**Eligibility**: A Council on Education for Public Health (CEPH) accredited school of public health or another public or nonprofit private institution accredited for the provision of graduate or specialized training in public health. | Regents of the University of California, Los Angeles | CA | $650,000 |
| | University of South Florida | FL | 650,000 |
| | Emory University | GA | 650,000 |
| | The Board of Trustees of the University of Illinois | IL | 650,000 |
| | University of Iowa | IA | 650,000 |
| | The Regents of the University of Michigan | MI | 650,000 |
| | Regents of the University of Minnesota | MN | 650,000 |
| | Board of Regents of the University of Nebraska, UNMC[a] | NE | 650,000 |
| | University of South Carolina | SC | 650,000 |
| | East Tennessee State University | TN | 650,000 |
| | University of Washington | WA | 650,000 |
| | Yale University[a] | CT | 649,998 |
| | University of Pittsburgh | PA | 649,995 |
| | University of Colorado Denver | CO | 649,990 |
| | University of Alabama at Birmingham[a] | AL | 649,981 |
| | Trustees of Boston University, BUMC | MA | 649,972 |
| | The Regents of the University of California | CA | 649,905 |
| | The University of Texas Health Science Center at Houston | TX | 649,819 |
| | The Research Foundation of SUNY | NY | 649,496 |
| | Board of Regents of the University of Wisconsin System | WI | 647,154 |
| | University of Florida[a] | FL | 645,158 |
| | Arizona Board of Regents | AZ | 645,038 |
| | UMDNJ-New Jersey-School of Public Health | NJ | 644,441 |
| | The University of Oklahoma Health Sciences Center | OK | 642,064 |
| | University of Puerto Rico Medical Sciences Campus | PR | 640,879 |
| | University of North Carolina at Chapel Hill | NC | 639,004 |
| | The University of Georgia | GA | 633,022 |
| | Trustees of Dartmouth College | NH | 619,090 |
| | University of Massachusetts Amherst[a] | MA | 614,589 |
| | University of Kentucky Research Foundation | KY | 610,781 |
| | Eastern Virginia Medical School | VA | 491,849 |
| | Indiana University | IN | 129,748 |
| | **Total (32 awards)** | | **$19,951,973** |

Source: GAO analysis of HHS information.

[a]Indicates new awards for five recipients, remainder are continuation awards.

## Activity: Advanced Nursing Education

The purpose of this activity is to build and enhance advanced nursing education programs, including grants to schools of nursing to accelerate the education of primary care advanced practice nurses.

- **Fiscal year 2010**: $31 million (26 grants in one funding announcement)

- **Fiscal year 2011**: None

**Table 66: FY 2010 Grants, Advanced Nursing Education**

| Announcement | Recipient | State | Award (dollars) |
|---|---|---|---|
| Advanced Nursing Education Expansion (HRSA-10-281)<br><br>**Purpose (award type)**: To increase the number of students enrolled full time in accredited primary care Nurse Practitioner and Nurse Midwifery programs and to accelerate the graduation of part time students in such programs by encouraging full time enrollment. The program provides master's, post master's, and, on a limited basis, doctor of nursing practice students with stipends, educational expenses, or other reasonable living expenses for $22,000 per year, for a maximum of two years per student, plus indirect costs. (New)<br><br>**Legislative Authority**: Section 811(a)(1) of the Public Health Service Act (42 U.S.C. 296j(a)(1), as amended by section 5308 of the Affordable Care Act (Pub. L. 111-148), and section 4002 of the Patient Protection and Affordable Care Act (Pub. L. 111-148).<br><br>**Eligibility**: Collegiate schools of nursing, academic health centers, and other private or public entities accredited by a national nursing accrediting agency recognized by the Secretary of the U.S. Department of Education that offer and have students enrolled in a primary care nurse practitioner program and/or an accredited nurse-midwifery program. | Florida State University | FL | $1,425,600 |
| | University of Illinois at Chicago/The Board of Trustees of the University of Illinois | IL | 1,425,600 |
| | Michigan State University | MI | 1,425,600 |
| | The University of Michigan-Flint | MI | 1,425,600 |
| | Daemen College | NY | 1,425,600 |
| | Pace University | NY | 1,425,600 |
| | Case Western Reserve Univ | OH | 1,425,600 |
| | Medical Univ of South Carolina | SC | 1,425,600 |
| | East Tennessee State University | TN | 1,425,600 |
| | University of Texas Health Science Center at San Antonio | TX | 1,425,600 |
| | Univ of Utah | UT | 1,425,600 |
| | The Pennsylvania State Univ | PA | 1,335,840 |
| | College of St. Scholastica | MN | 1,330,560 |
| | Wayne State University | MI | 1,320,000 |
| | Oregon Health & Science University | OR | 1,283,040 |
| | Duke Univ School of Nursing | NC | 1,276,000 |
| | Shenandoah Univ | VA | 1,188,000 |
| | Western Univ of Health Sciences | CA | 1,056,000 |
| | Trustees of the Univ of Pennsylvania | PA | 950,400 |
| | West Virginia University Rsch Corporation | WV | 950,400 |
| | Georgia State Univ Research Foundation, Inc. | GA | 831,600 |
| | Rutgers, The State University | NJ | 807,840 |
| | Univ of Oklahoma Health Sciences Center | OK | 807,840 |
| | Univ of Massachusetts Medical School | MA | 760,816 |

| Announcement | Recipient | State | Award (dollars) |
|---|---|---|---|
| | Univ of Detroit Mercy | MI | 760,320 |
| | University of Miami | FL | 704,000 |
| | **Total (26 awards)** | | **$31,044,256** |

Source: GAO analysis of HHS information.

## Activity: Nurse Managed Care Centers

The purpose of this activity is to support nurse managed clinics which improve access to primary care, enhance nursing practice by increasing the number of clinical teaching sites for primary care and community health nursing students, and develop electronic processes for establishing effective patient and workforce data collection systems.

- **Fiscal year 2010**: $14.8 million (10 grants in one funding announcement)

- **Fiscal year 2011**: None

## Table 67: FY 2010 Grants, Nurse Managed Care Centers

| Announcement | Recipient | State | Award (dollars) |
|---|---|---|---|
| Nurse Managed Health Clinics (HRSA-10-282) | Fair Haven Community Health Clinic, Inc. | CT | $1,500,000 |
| **Purpose (award type):** To support the development and operation of Nurse-Managed Health Clinics (NMHC) to: (1) improve access to comprehensive primary health care and/or wellness services (disease prevention and health promotion) across the lifespan, (2) provide services in medically underserved areas and/or for vulnerable populations; (3) serve as clinical training sites for students in primary care and specifically, enhance nursing practice by increasing the number of structured clinical teaching sites for primary and community health graduate nursing students; and (4) establish or enhance electronic processes for establishing effective patient and workforce data collection systems. (New) | University of Mississippi Medical Center | MS | 1,500,000 |
| | The University of Texas Medical Branch at Galveston | TX | 1,500,000 |
| | University of Illinois at Chicago/The Board of Trustees of the University of Illinois | IL | 1,499,995 |
| | Regents of the Univ of Michigan | MI | 1,498,577 |
| | University of Colorado, Denver | CO | 1,498,206 |
| | The Regents of the University of California, San Francisco | CA | 1,497,320 |
| | St. Mary's Health Wagon, Inc. | VA | 1,493,634 |
| | Tides Center–Women's Community Clinic | CA | 1,459,366 |
| | East Tennessee State University | TN | 1,400,998 |
| **Legislative Authority**: Section 330A-1 of the Public Health Service Act (42 U.S.C. 254c-1a) as added by Section 5208 of the Patient Protection and Affordable Care Act (Pub. L. 111-148), and section 4002 of the Patient Protection and Affordable Care Act (Pub. L. 111-148). | **Total (10 awards)** | | **$14,848,096** |
| **Eligibility**: Nurse-managed health clinics (NMHC) that are associated with an accredited school, college, university, or department of nursing, federally qualified health center or independent nonprofit health or social services agency. Applicants must provide primary care or wellness services to vulnerable and/or underserved populations. | | | |

Source: GAO analysis of HHS information.

**Activity**: State Health Workforce Development Grants for Primary Care

The purpose of this activity is to provide support to states in expanding their health care workforce by enabling state partnerships (generally the State Workforce Investment Board) to complete comprehensive planning and to carry out activities leading to coherent and comprehensive health care workforce development strategies at the state and local levels, with particular emphasis on primary care.

- **Fiscal Year 2010**: $5.6 million (26 grants in two funding announcements)

- **Fiscal Year 2011**: None

**Table 68: FY 2010 Grants, State Health Workforce Development Grants for Primary Care**

| Announcements (2) | Recipient | State | Award (dollars) |
|---|---|---|---|
| 1. State Health Care Workforce Planning Grants (HRSA-10-284)<br><br>**Purpose (award type)**: To enable State partnerships to complete comprehensive health care workforce development planning to address current and projected workforce demands within the State. (New)<br><br>**Legislative Authority**: Section 5102 of the Affordable Care Act; and section 4002 of the Patient Protection and Affordable Care Act, Public Law 111-148.<br><br>**Eligibility**: Limited to eligible State partnerships (generally a State Workforce Investment Board) that includes, or modifies the members to include, at least one representative from each of the following: health care employer, labor organization, a public 2-year institution of higher education, a public 4-year institution of higher education, the recognized State federation of labor, the State public secondary education agency, the State P-16 or P-20 Council (statewide assemblies of education, business, and community leaders charged with developing strategies to better coordinate, integrate, and improve education for preschool through college students), if such a council exists, and a philanthropic organization that is actively engaged in providing learning, mentoring, and work opportunities to recruit, educate, and train individuals for, and retain individuals in, careers in health care and related industries. | California Department of Employment Development | CA | $150,000 |
| | Colorado Department of Public Health and Environment | CO | 150,000 |
| | Connecticut Employment & Training Commission | CT | 150,000 |
| | Hawaii Department of Labor and Industrial Relations | HI | 150,000 |
| | Idaho Department of Labor | ID | 150,000 |
| | Kansas Department of Commerce | KS | 150,000 |
| | Maine Jobs Council | ME | 150,000 |
| | Maryland Governor's Workforce Investment Board | MD | 150,000 |
| | Montana State University | MT | 150,000 |
| | NJ Department of Labor and Workforce | NJ | 150,000 |
| | New Mexico Department of Labor | NM | 150,000 |
| | New York State Department of Labor | NY | 150,000 |
| | University of North Dakota | ND | 150,000 |
| | Alaska Department of Labor And Workforce Development, ESD | AK | 150,000 |
| | State of Ohio – Department of Health | OH | 150,000 |
| | Pennsylvania Department of Labor & Industry | PA | 150,000 |
| | University of Wisconsin –Madison | WI | 150,000 |
| | Nevada Dept of Employment, Training, and Rehabilitation | NV | 149,999 |
| | MN Department of Employment and Economic Development | MN | 149,599 |
| | Wyoming Department of Workforce Services | WY | 149,396 |
| | Commonwealth Corporation | MA | 149,271 |
| | District of Columbia Department of Employment Services | DC | 149,250 |
| | North Carolina Department of Commerce Division of Workforce Development | NC | 144,595 |
| | University of Vermont | VT | 131,786 |
| | South Carolina Department of Employment and Workforce | SC | 114,604 |
| | **Total (25 awards)** | | **$3,688,500** |

| Announcements (2) | Recipient | State | Award (dollars) |
|---|---|---|---|
| 2. State Health Care Workforce Implementation Grants (HRSA-10-285) | Virginia State Department of Health | VA | $1,935,137 |
| | **Total (1 award)** | | **$1,935,137** |

**Purpose (award type)**: To enable State partnerships to implement workforce development plans or carry out activities as defined by the State application in order to address current and projected workforce demands within the State.(New)

**Legislative Authority**: Section 5102 of the Affordable Care Act; and section 4002 of the Patient Protection and Affordable Care Act, Public Law 111-148.

**Eligibility**: A State partnership shall have (1) received a planning grant as specified under subsection c of Section 5102, P.L. 111-148 and completed all requirements of such grant; or (2) completed a satisfactory application, including a plan to coordinate with required partners and complete the required activities during the two year period of the implementation grant.

Source: GAO analysis of HHS information.

**Activity**: HRSA Healthy Weight Collaborative and Activities

The purpose of this activity is to integrate primary care, public health, and the community by using quality improvement science to identify, test, and disseminate evidence-based interventions to prevent and treat obesity in children and families.

- **Fiscal year 2010**: $5.0 million (one grant in one funding announcement)

- **Fiscal year 2011**: None

**Table 69: FY 2010 Grants, HRSA Healthy Weight Collaborative**

| Announcement | Recipient | State | Award (dollars) |
|---|---|---|---|
| Prevention Center For Healthy Weight (HRSA-10-303) | National Initiative For Children's Healthcare Quality | MA | $4,983,638 |
| | **Total (1 award)** | | **$4,983,638** |

**Purpose (award type)**: To support a Prevention Center for Healthy Weight (PC) to plan, implement, and manage a nation-wide Healthy Weight Collaborative (HWC) as well as recruit and support communities and teams participating in the HWC. The PC will also serve as a gateway to quality information on the prevention and treatment of overweight and obesity in the context of integration of public and community health and primary care. (New)

**Legislative Authority**: Title V, Section 501(a)(2) Social Security Act (42 U.S.C. 701) and Section 4002 of the Patient Protection and Affordable Care Act (P.L. 111-148).

**Eligibility**: Any public or private nonprofit entity, including state and local government agencies, institutions of higher education, and an Indian tribe or tribal organization. Applicants must have at least four years experience in the fields of quality management, quality improvement, developing and disseminating informational materials, and providing training or technical assistance related to the prevention and treatment of overweight and obesity on a national level. The applicant should have experience working with public health, community-based organizations, primary care, behavioral health, and academic institutions in addressing these concerns. The Prevention Center may be a consortium of organizations composed of more than one eligible entity, but only one entity can be the official applicant for funding. All other organizations are members of the consortium or partnership.

Source: GAO analysis of HHS information.

## Activity: Nutrition, Physical Activity, and Screen Time Standards in Child Care Settings

The purpose of this activity is to enhance the quality of out-of-home child care by supporting the state and local health departments, early care and education regulatory agencies, early care and education providers, and parents in their efforts to identify and promote healthy and safe early care.

- **Fiscal year 2010**: $0.2 million (one grant in one funding announcement)

- **Fiscal year 2011**: None

**Table 70: FY 2010 Grant, Nutrition, Physical Activity, and Screen Time Standards in Child Care Settings**

| Announcement | Recipient | State | Award (dollars) |
|---|---|---|---|
| National Resource Center for Health and Safety in Child Care Settings (HRSA-05-058) | University of Colorado, Denver, College of Nursing | CO | $249,000 |
| | **Total (1 award)** | | **$249,000** |

**Purpose (award type)**: The National Resource Center (NRC) In partnership with national experts (American Academy of Pediatrics and American Public Health Association), coordinates the development, updating and promotion of voluntary national evidence-based health and safety standards for child care programs—commonly referred to as Caring for Our Children. (Supplement)

**Legislative Authority**: Title V, Section 501(a)(2-3) Social Security Act (42 U.S.C. 701) and Section 4002 of the Patient Protection and Affordable Care Act (P.L. 111-148).

**Eligibility**: Supplemental funding to the National Resource Center for Health and Safety in Child Care, University of Colorado, Denver, College of Nursing.

Source: GAO analysis of HHS information.

# Appendix IV: Office of the Secretary—Prevention and Public Health Fund Awards by Activity

This appendix presents information on awards made by the Office of the Secretary (OS) for Prevention and Public Health Fund (PPHF) activities with funds allocated and transferred from the PPHF for fiscal years (FY) 2010 and 2011. For each OS activity that received PPHF funding, tables 71 through 77 summarize information on awards made with those funds through grants and contracts for each fiscal year.[1] Award information was provided by HHS's Assistant Secretary for Financial Resources and OS officials.

The information presented in this appendix, including the purpose of the PPHF-funded activity, was obtained from HHS. Due to the large number of awards, we did not edit the award recipient information to correct typographical or grammatical errors, or clarify the information provided. In general, we reprinted the abbreviations and acronyms provided by HHS. Totals in this appendix (reported obligations) may not match—for example, they may be lower than—the amounts in table 2 (reported allocations). According to HHS officials, to carry out an activity, an agency may incur administrative expenses, including an agency's internal costs associated with managing and overseeing grants and contracts, not reflected in award amounts. Further, to the extent that an appropriation has not identified a particular amount for a specific activity, an agency may reallocate unobligated funds from that activity to another during the course of a fiscal year.

**Activity**: Obesity Media Activities

The purpose of this activity is to develop and execute innovative communication campaigns, including both print and online materials development for anti-obesity and healthy lifestyle initiatives.

- **Fiscal year 2010**: $9.1 million (one contract)

- **Fiscal year 2011**: $8.6 million (two contracts)

---

[1]The tables present information on cooperative agreements with grants, and include information on interagency agreements with contracts.

Appendix IV: Office of the Secretary—
Prevention and Public Health Fund Awards by
Activity

**Table 71: FY 2010 Contracts, Obesity Media Activities**

| Recipient | Purpose | State | Award (dollars) |
|---|---|---|---|
| Oglivy Public Relations | Develop strategic outreach plans | NY | $9,100,000 |
| Total (1 award) | | | **$9,100,000** |

Source: GAO analysis of HHS information.

**Table 72: FY 2011 Contracts, Obesity Media Activities**

| Recipient | Purpose | State | Award (dollars) |
|---|---|---|---|
| Oglivy Public Relations | Public awareness campaigns | NY | $5,993,740 |
| Ad Council | Public awareness campaigns | NY | 2,650,000 |
| Total (2 awards) | | | **$8,643,740** |

Source: GAO analysis of HHS information.

## Activity: Tobacco Prevention Media

The purpose of this activity is to launch a mass-media countermarketing campaign to prevent youth initiation, promote cessation among adults, and change social norms, using social media initiatives, a website, and smart phone applications.

- **Fiscal year 2010**: None

- **Fiscal year 2011**: $10.1 million (12 contracts)

Appendix IV: Office of the Secretary—
Prevention and Public Health Fund Awards by
Activity

**Table 73: FY 2011 Contracts, Tobacco Prevention Media**

| Recipient | Purpose | State | Award (dollars) |
|---|---|---|---|
| PlowShare Group Inc | Smoking Cessation campaign | CT | $4,000,000 |
| Aquilent | Web development | MD | 2,052,116 |
| Matthews Media Group | Smoking Cessation campaign | MD | 2,000,000 |
| Aquilent | Web development | MD | 494,224 |
| American Independent Media | Studio activities in support of tobacco related messaging | MD | 425,000 |
| Communication Training Analysis Corporation | Research and database | VA | 298,939 |
| Communication Training Analysis Corporation | Research and database | VA | 229,960 |
| Aquilent | Web development | MD | 221,064 |
| Intelligent Enterprise Solutions | Develop engine to syndicate content | MD | 200,000 |
| Interagency Agreement with OASH | Content support | | 125,000 |
| PSC | Various processing fees | | 21,943 |
| Web Training | Web training | | 3,500 |
| **Total (12 awards)** | | | **$10,071,746** |

Source: GAO analysis of HHS information.

## Activity: National Prevention, Health Promotion, and Public Health Council Planning

The purpose of this activity is to support the National Prevention Council, including a national conference that will bring together individuals, agencies, organizations, and programs that are putting into practice activities that will advance prevention per the Healthy People 2020 initiative.

- **Fiscal year 2010**: $1.1 million (one grant for $0.1 million[2] and three contracts totaling $1.0 million)

- **Fiscal year 2011**: None

[2]HHS did not provide a funding announcement for this award. According to HHS officials, OS awarded $138,000 to the Association for Prevention Teaching Workshop for fiscal year 2010.

Appendix IV: Office of the Secretary—
Prevention and Public Health Fund Awards by
Activity

**Table 74: FY 2010 Contracts, National Prevention, Health Promotion, and Public Health Council Planning**

| Recipient | Purpose | State | Award (dollars) |
|---|---|---|---|
| IQ Solutions, Inc. | Contracts to support strategic planning within the Office of Public Health and Science, such as support for the National Prevention, Health Promotion, and Public Health Council and Advisory Group in section 4001 of the Affordable Care Act. | | $620,000 |
| American Institutes For Research | | | 66,000 |
| National Opinion Research Center | | | 300,000 |
| **Total (3 awards)** | | | **$986,000** |

Source: GAO analysis of HHS information.

## Activity: President's Council on Fitness, Sports, and Nutrition

The purpose of this activity is to coordinate obesity activities, including the Let's Move Ambassador Program; the President's Active Lifestyle Awards Program; the Youth Empowerment Program, and support for a Leadership Development Series for the Council.

- **Fiscal year 2010**: $0.8 million (two contracts)

- **Fiscal year 2011**: None

**Table 75: FY 2010 Contracts, President's Council on Fitness, Sports, and Nutrition**

| Recipient | Purpose | State | Award (dollars) |
|---|---|---|---|
| National Initiative on Physical Fitness for Children and Youth with Disabilities (OPHS-10-239) | Interagency agreements to coordinate obesity, including the Let's Move Ambassador Program; the President's Active Lifestyle Awards Program; the Youth Empowerment Program, and support for a Leadership Development Series for the Council. | | $500,000 |
| Research Participation Program (OPHS-10-228) | | | 292,000 |
| **Total (2 awards)** | | | **$792,000** |

Source: GAO analysis of HHS information.

## Activity: Tobacco Cessation

The purpose of this activity is to implement tobacco cessation activities, such as reducing tobacco use among low social economic status women of childbearing age, reducing the impact of tobacco use on their children, and other outreach efforts.

- **Fiscal year 2010**: $0.7 million (three contracts)

- **Fiscal year 2011**: None

Appendix IV: Office of the Secretary—
Prevention and Public Health Fund Awards by
Activity

**Table 76: FY 2010 Contracts, Tobacco Cessation**

| Recipient | Purpose | State | Award (dollars) |
|---|---|---|---|
| Tobacco and Young, Low-SES Women Federal Collaboration Smoking Cessation and Prevention Program (OPHS-10-213) | Contract and interagency agreements to implement tobacco cessation activities, such as reducing tobacco use among low social economic status women of childbearing age, reducing the impact of tobacco use on their children, and other outreach efforts. | | $285,000 |
| American Institutes for Research | | | 226,000 |
| LSES Women and Tobacco Collaborative Demonstration Project (OPHS-10-231) | | | 150,000 |
| **Total (3 awards)** | | | **$661,000** |

Source: GAO analysis of HHS information.

## Activity: Healthy Living Innovations Awards

The purpose of this activity is to create a public challenge project that would address three health promotion areas: healthy weight, physical activity, and nutrition. Project funds were used to develop the website, market the challenge, coordinate the review process for 250 applications, develop a monthly report on the website analytics, and manage the logistics of bringing the challenge winners to Washington, D.C. to received an award (plaques) and present on their projects at a national conference. The contractor also developed a final report documenting the process and highlighting areas of improvement.

- **Fiscal year 2010**: $0.1 million (one contract)

- **Fiscal year 2011**: None

**Table 77: FY 2010 Contract, Healthy Living Innovations Awards**

| Recipient | Purpose | State | Award (dollars) |
|---|---|---|---|
| NORC at the University of Chicago | Administer awards program | MD | $100,000 |
| **Total (1 award)** | | | **$100,000** |

Source: GAO analysis of HHS information.

# Appendix V: Substance Abuse and Mental Health Services Administration—Prevention and Public Health Fund Awards by Activity

This appendix presents information on awards made by the Substance Abuse and Mental Health Services Administration (SAMHSA) for Prevention and Public Health Fund (PPHF) activities with funds allocated and transferred from the PPHF for fiscal years (FY) 2010 and 2011. For each SAMHSA activity that received PPHF funding, tables 78 through 83 summarize information on awards made with those funds through grants and contracts for each fiscal year.[1] Award information was provided by HHS's Assistant Secretary for Financial Resources, SAMHSA, or reported in the funding opportunity announcements (FOA) HHS identified as being associated with the activity and awards.

The information presented in this appendix, including the purpose of the PPHF-funded activity, was obtained from HHS. Due to the large number of awards, we did not edit the award recipient information to correct typographical or grammatical errors, or clarify the information provided. In general, we reprinted the abbreviations and acronyms provided by HHS and the legislative authority cited in the FOA or otherwise provided by HHS. We did not independently verify the legislative authority. Totals in this appendix (reported obligations) may not match—for example, they may be lower than—the amounts in table 2 (reported allocations). According to HHS officials, to carry out an activity, an agency may incur administrative expenses, including an agency's internal costs associated with managing and overseeing grants and contracts, not reflected in award amounts. Further, to the extent that an appropriation has not identified a particular amount for a specific activity, an agency may reallocate unobligated funds from that activity to another during the course of a fiscal year.

Activity: Primary and Behavioral Health Care Integration

The purpose of this activity is to improve the physical health status of people with serious mental illnesses by supporting communities to coordinate and integrate primary care services in community mental health and other community-based behavioral health settings.

---

[1]The tables present information on cooperative agreements with grants, and include information on interagency agreements with contracts.

- **Fiscal year 2010**: $20.0 million (35 grants in two funding announcements)

- **Fiscal year 2011**: $35.0 million (43 grants in two funding announcements)

**Table 78: FY 2010 Grants, Primary and Behavioral Health Care Integration**

| Announcements (2) | Recipient | State | Award (dollars) |
|---|---|---|---|
| 1. Grants for Primary and Behavioral Health Care Integration (SM-09-011)<br><br>**Purpose (award type):** To improve the overall wellness and physical health status of people with serious mental illnesses by making available coordinated primary care services in community mental health and other community-based behavioral health settings. SAMHSA expects that people with serious mental illnesses will show improvement in their physical health status through participation in the programs associated with this grant. PBHCI also includes a focus on providing wellness education and support services. This grant program supports SAMHSA's Pledge for Wellness 10 by 10 Campaign to prevent and reduce early mortality among people with mental illness by 10 years over the next 10 years. It is projected that better coordination and integration of primary and behavioral health care should lead to outcomes such as improved access to primary care services; improved prevention, early identification and intervention to avoid serious health issues including chronic diseases; enhanced capacity to holistically serve those with mental and/or substance use disorders; and better overall health status of clients. (New)<br><br>**Legislative Authority:** Section 520A of the Public Health Service Act, as amended.<br><br>**Eligibility:** Limited to publicly funded community mental health and other community-based behavioral health agencies. For the purposes of this announcement, community mental health and other behavioral health agencies are defined as the following: (1) an entity that meets applicable licensing or certification requirements in the State in which it is located; and (2) provides outpatient mental health and/or other behavioral health services for individuals with serious mental illness. | Community Mental Health Affiliates, Inc. | CT | $496,863 |
| | Asian Community Mental Health Board | CA | 496,863 |
| | Glenn County Health Services Agency | CA | 496,863 |
| | Apalachee Center, Inc. | FL | 496,863 |
| | Coastal Behavioral Healthcare, Inc. | FL | 496,863 |
| | Miami Behavioral Health Center, Inc. | FL | 496,863 |
| | Heritage Behavioral Health Center, Inc. | IL | 496,863 |
| | St. Barnabas Hospital | NY | 496,863 |
| | North Oklahoma County Mental Health Center | OK | 496,863 |
| | Asian Counseling and Referral Services | WA | 496,863 |
| | Tarzana Treatment Centers, Inc. | CA | 496,862 |
| | Community Rehab Center (CRC), Inc. | FL | 496,862 |
| | LifeStream Behavioral Center | FL | 496,862 |
| | Washtenaw Community Health Organization | MI | 496,862 |
| | Catholic Charities, Diocese of Trenton | NJ | 496,862 |
| | Weber Human Services | UT | 496,862 |
| | Cobb County Community Services Board | GA | 496,825 |
| | Community Health and Counseling Services | ME | 496,820 |
| | Kent Center for Human and Organizational Development | RI | 496,636 |
| | Postgraduate Center for Mental Health | NY | 496,372 |
| | County of San Mateo | CA | 496,307 |
| | Bronx Lebanon Hospital Center | NY | 496,135 |
| | Adult and Child Mental Health Center, Inc. | IN | 495,189 |
| | Austin Travis County MH/MR Center | TX | 494,900 |
| | Greater Cincinnati Behavioral Health Services | OH | 492,511 |
| | Family Services, Inc. | MD | 490,868 |
| | Downtown Emergency Services Center | WA | 482,394 |
| | Horizon House, Inc. | PA | 481,562 |
| | South Carolina Department of Mental Health | SC | 471,654 |

| Announcements (2) | Recipient | State | Award (dollars) |
|---|---|---|---|
| | Community Healthlink, Inc. | MA | 460,690 |
| | Lakeside Behavioral Healthcare, Inc. | FL | 448,343 |
| | Prestera Center for Mental Health Services, Inc. | WV | 438,513 |
| | Trilogy, Inc. | IL | 421,263 |
| | Alaska Island Community Services | AK | 296,836 |
| | **Total (34 awards)** | | **$16,403,620** |
| 2. Training and Technical Assistance Center for Primary and Behavioral Health Care Integration (TTA-PBHCI) (SM-10-011) | National Council for Community Behavioral Healthcare | DC | $3,596,380 |
| | **Total (1 award)** | | **$3,596,380** |

2. **Training and Technical Assistance Center for Primary and Behavioral Health Care Integration (TTA-PBHCI) (SM-10-011)**

**Purpose (award type)**: To provide technical assistance support for up to 30 additional grantees, support a coordinated approach to address workforce development issues affecting the behavioral health service delivery community, and promote the training and use of behavioral health screening, brief intervention and referral for treatment in primary care settings. (New)

**Legislative Authority**: Section 520A (SAMHSA) and 330(1) (HRSA) of the Public Health Service Act, as amended.

**Eligibility**: Eligible applicants are domestic public and private nonprofit entities. For example, State and local governments, federally recognized American Indian/Alaska Native Tribes and tribal organizations, urban Indian organizations, public or private universities and colleges; and community- and faith-based organizations may apply. Tribal organization means the recognized body of any AI/AN Tribe; any legally established organization of American Indians/Alaska Natives which is controlled, sanctioned, or chartered by such governing body or which is democratically elected by the adult members of the Indian community to be served by such organization and which includes the maximum participation of American Indians/Alaska Natives in all phases of its activities. Consortia of tribal organizations are eligible to apply, but each participating entity must indicate its approval.

Source: GAO analysis of HHS information.

**Table 79: FY 2011 Grants, Primary and Behavioral Health Care Integration**

| Announcements (2) | Recipient | State | Award (dollars) |
|---|---|---|---|
| 1. Grants for Primary and Behavioral Health Care Integration (SM-09-011) | Capital Area Human Services District[a] | LA | $1,893,939 |
| | Catholic Charities of Santa Clara County[a] | CA | 1,893,939 |
| **Purpose (award type)**: To improve the overall wellness and physical health status of people with serious mental illnesses by making available coordinated primary care services in community mental health and other community-based behavioral health settings. (New and Continuation) | Highline West Seattle Mental Health[a] | WA | 1,893,939 |
| | Norfolk Community Services Board[a] | VA | 1,893,939 |
| | San Francisco Department of Public Health[a] | CA | 1,893,939 |
| | SouthCentral Foundation[a] | AK | 1,893,939 |
| **Legislative Authority**: Section 520A of the Public Health Service Act, as amended. | Community Support Services Inc.[a] | OH | 1,836,954 |
| | Health and Hospital Corp of Marion County[a] | IN | 1,834,412 |
| **Eligibility**: Limited to publicly funded community mental health and other community-based behavioral health agencies. For the purposes of this announcement, community mental health and other behavioral health agencies are defined as the following: (1) an entity that meets applicable licensing or certification requirements in the State in which it is located; and (2) provides outpatient mental health and/or other behavioral health services for individuals with serious mental illness. | Apalachee Center, Inc. | FL | 500,000 |
| | Asian Community Mental Health Board | CA | 500,000 |
| | Asian Counseling and Referral Services | WA | 500,000 |
| | Catholic Charities, Diocese of Trenton | NJ | 500,000 |
| | Coastal Behavioral Healthcare, Inc. | FL | 500,000 |
| | Community Mental Health Affiliates, Inc. | CT | 500,000 |
| | Community Rehab Center (CRC), Inc. | FL | 500,000 |
| | Family Services, Inc. | MD | 500,000 |
| | Glenn County Health Services Agency | CA | 500,000 |
| | Heritage Behavioral Health Center, Inc. | IL | 500,000 |
| | LifeStream Behavioral Center | FL | 500,000 |
| | Miami Behavioral Health Center, Inc. | FL | 500,000 |
| | North Oklahoma County Mental Health Center | OK | 500,000 |
| | Tarzana Treatment Centers, Inc. | CA | 500,000 |
| | Washtenaw Community Health Organization | MI | 500,000 |
| | Community Health and Counseling Services | ME | 499,957 |
| | Postgraduate Center for Mental Health | NY | 499,510 |
| | County of San Mateo | CA | 499,444 |
| | Bronx Lebanon Hospital Center | NY | 499,272 |
| | Cobb County Community Services Board | GA | 498,825 |
| | Adult and Child Mental Health Center, Inc. | IN | 498,061 |
| | Austin Travis County MH/MR Center | TX | 498,037 |
| | St. Barnabas Hospital | NY | 496,863 |
| | Kent Center for Human and Organizational Development | RI | 492,281 |
| | Downtown Emergency Services Center | WA | 485,531 |
| | Community Healthlink, Inc. | MA | 484,964 |

| Announcements (2) | Recipient | State | Award (dollars) |
|---|---|---|---|
| | Greater Cincinnati Behavioral Health Services | OH | 483,637 |
| | Prestera Center for Mental Health Services, Inc. | WV | 481,091 |
| | South Carolina Department of Mental Health | SC | 478,049 |
| | Horizon House, Inc. | PA | 467,609 |
| | Lakeside Behavioral Healthcare, Inc. | FL | 455,033 |
| | Trilogy, Inc. | IL | 387,218 |
| | Weber Human Services | UT | 365,000 |
| | Alaska Island Community Services | AK | 300,000 |
| | **Total (42 awards)** | | **$31,405,382** |
| 2. Continuation to the Training and Technical Assistance Center for Primary and Behavioral Health Care Integration (TTA-PBHCI)(SM-10-011) | National Council for Community Behavioral Healthcare | DC | $3,594,045 |
| **Purpose (award type)**: To provide technical assistance support for a coordinated approach to address workforce development issues affecting the behavioral health service delivery community, and promote the training and use of behavioral health screening, brief intervention and referral for treatment in primary care settings. (Continuation) | **Total (1 award)** | | **$3,594,045** |
| **Legislative Authority**: Section 520A (SAMHSA) and 330(1) (HRSA) of the Public Health Service Act, as amended. | | | |
| **Eligibility**: Limited to the National Council for Community Behavioral Healthcare (NCCBH), based on the Council's expertise and relationship with the PBHCI grantees. | | | |

Source: GAO analysis of HHS information.

[a]Indicates new awards for eight recipients, remainder are continuation awards.

## Activity: Screening, Brief Intervention, and Referral to Treatment

The purpose of this activity is to implement screening, brief intervention, and referral to treatment services for adults in primary care and community health settings, for substance misuse and substance use disorders. This program is designed to expand/enhance the state and tribal continuum of care for substance misuse services and reduce alcohol and drug consumption and its negative health impact; increase abstinence and reduce costly health care utilization; and promote sustainability and behavioral health information technology.

- **Fiscal year 2010**: None

- **Fiscal year 2011**: $25.0 million (three grants in one funding announcement)

**Table 80: FY 2011 Grants, Screening, Brief Intervention, and Referral to Treatment**

| Announcement | Recipient | State | Award (dollars) |
|---|---|---|---|
| Cooperative Agreements for Screening, Brief Intervention and Referral to Treatment (SBIRT) (TI-11-005) | North Carolina Department of Health and Human Services | NC | $8,330,000 |
| | State of Connecticut | CT | 8,330,000 |
| | State of Indiana | IN | 8,329,906 |
| **Purpose (award type)**: To expand/enhance the State/Tribe's continuum of care to include universal, adult SBIRT services in primary care and a mix of other community settings (e.g., health centers, nursing homes, university health centers, employee assistance and job training sites, hospitals, emergency departments, office-based practices and Military, Reserve and Guard units) and supports clinically appropriate services for persons at risk (asymptomatic) for, or diagnosed with, a substance use disorder (SUD). It also seeks to identify and sustain systems and policy changes to increase access to treatment in generalist and specialist settings. (New) | **Total (3 awards)** | | **$24,989,906** |
| **Legislative Authority**: Section 509 of the Public Health Service Act, as amended. | | | |
| **Eligibility**: The immediate office of the Chief Executive (e.g., Governor) in the States, Territories, and District of Columbia; and the highest ranking official and/or the duly authorized official of a federally recognized American Indian/Alaska Native Tribe or tribal organization. | | | |

Source: GAO analysis of HHS information.

### Activity: SAMHSA Health Surveillance

The purpose of this activity is to support a number of federal, state, local, and tribal governments, as well as researchers and nongovernmental organizations, to develop timely and credible data and statistical information to improve the quality and outcomes of services provided to individuals, families, communities, and tribal communities.

- **Fiscal year 2010**: None

- **Fiscal year 2011**: $17.9 million (seven contracts)

**Table 81: FY 2011 Contracts, SAMHSA Health Surveillance**

| Recipient | Purpose | State | Award (dollars) |
|---|---|---|---|
| Westat | DAWN Operations and Emergency room data collection | MD | $8,804,701 |
| Manila Consulting | Expansion of NREPP | VA | 3,547,794 |
| Synectics for Management Decisions | Expansion of Mental Health inventories | VA | 2,400,704 |
| RTI International | DAWN Analysis contract modification | NC | 1,503,561 |
| The Mitre Corporation | MITRE FFRDC | VA | 757,272 |
| RTI International | Analysis on NSDUH data system | NC | 690,412 |
| Manila Consulting | SAMHSA Data Users Conference on prevention research | VA | 200,000 |
| **Total (7 awards)** | | | **$17,904,444** |

Source: GAO analysis of HHS information.

## Activity: Suicide Prevention

The Garrett Lee Smith (GLS) Memorial Act authorizes SAMHSA to
manage two significant youth suicide prevention programs and a resource
center. The GLS State/Tribal Youth Suicide Prevention and Early
Intervention Grant Program supports the development and
implementation of youth suicide prevention and early intervention
strategies involving public-private collaborations among youth-serving
institutions. The GLS Campus Suicide Prevention program provides
funding to institutions of higher education to prevent suicide and suicide
attempts. The Suicide Prevention Resource Center (SPRC) develops
effective strategies and best practices to ensure the field has access to
the most crucial information.

- **Fiscal year 2010**: None

- **Fiscal year 2011**: $10.1 million (11 grants in four funding
  announcements totaling $10.0 million and one contract for
  $0.1 million)

**Table 82: FY 2011 Grants, Suicide Prevention**

| Announcements (4) | Recipient | State | Award (dollars) |
|---|---|---|---|
| 1.  State and Tribal Youth Suicide Prevention Grants (SM-11-001)<br><br>**Purpose (award type)**: To support States and tribes in developing and implementing statewide and/or tribal youth suicide prevention and early intervention strategies, grounded in public/private collaboration. Such efforts must involve public/private collaboration among youth serving institutions and agencies and should include schools, educational institutions, juvenile justice systems, foster care systems, substance abuse and mental health programs, and other child and youth supporting organizations. (New)<br><br>**Legislative Authority**: The Garrett Lee Smith Memorial Act (Section 520E-1 of the Public Health Service Act, as amended).<br><br>**Eligibility**: (1) States (Including D.C. and the Territories); (2) Federally recognized Indian tribes, tribal organizations (as defined in the Indian Self-Determination and Educational Assistance Act), or urban Indian organizations (as defined in the Indian Health Care Improvement Act) that are actively involved in the development and continuation of a tribal youth suicide early intervention and prevention strategy; and (3) Public or private non-profit organizations designated by a State, federally recognized Indian tribe, tribal organization, or urban Indian organization, to develop or direct the State/tribal-sponsored youth suicide prevention and early intervention strategy. | Pueblo of San Felipe - GLS States | NM | $1,440,000 |
| | Muscogee Creek Nation - GLS States | OK | 1,440,000 |
| | Native American Rehabilitation Assn - GLS States | OR | 1,440,000 |
| | Tohono O'Odham Nation - GLS States | AZ | 1,440,000 |
| | **Total (4 awards)** | | **$5,760,000** |
| 2.  Campus Suicide Prevention Grants (SM-11-002)<br><br>**Purpose (award type)**: To assist colleges and universities in their efforts to prevent suicide attempts and completions and to enhance services for students with mental and behavioral health problems, such as depression and substance use/abuse that put them at risk for suicide and suicide attempts. (New)<br><br>**Legislative Authority**: The Garrett Lee Smith Memorial Act (Section 520E-2 of the Public Health Service Act, as amended).<br><br>**Eligibility**: Limited to institutions of higher education as a statutory requirement (per Section 520E-2 of the Public Health Service Act, as amended). Applicants from both public and private institutions may apply, including State universities, private four-year colleges and universities (including those with religious affiliations), Minority Serving Institutions of higher learning, and community colleges. Entities that have previously been awarded a Campus Suicide Prevention Grant are not eligible. SAMHSA is further limiting the eligibility to applicants who have not previously received an award in order to allow for a broader distribution of the limited funds across campuses and universities. | University of Puerto Rico Rio Piedras - GLS Campus | PR | $306,000 |
| | Thomas Jefferson University - GLS Campus | PA | 306,000 |
| | University of Arizona - GLS Campus | AZ | 306,000 |
| | University of Alaska Anchorage - GLS Campus | AL | 306,000 |
| | Jackson State University - GLS Campus | MS | 306,000 |
| | **Total (5 awards)** | | **$1,530,000** |

| Announcements (4) | Recipient | State | Award (dollars) |
|---|---|---|---|
| 3. Program Supplement for the National Suicide Prevention Lifeline (SM-11-003) | Link2Health Solutions, Inc. - Suicide Hotline Supplement | NY | $1,705,000 |
| **Purpose (award type)**: To expand/enhance grant activities funded under the Cooperative Agreement for Networking, Certifying, and Training Suicide Prevention Hotlines grant announcement. Supplemental funding is being provided as a result of increased demand and challenges posed by the current economic environment. (Supplement) | **Total (1 award)** | | **$1,705,000** |
| **Legislative Authority**: Section 520A of the Public Health Service Act, as amended. | | | |
| **Eligibility**: Limited to the current grantee, Link2Health Solutions, Inc.. The grantee was awarded the cooperative agreement following a competitive application process. | | | |
| 4. Program Supplement for the Suicide Prevention Resource Center (SPRC) (SM-11-014) | Education Development Center, Inc. | MA | $999,993 |
| **Purpose (award type)**: To expand and enhance grant activities funded under the Suicide Prevention Resource Center (SPRC) grant announcement. This one-year supplement to the SPRC is to expand and enhance the level of support provided to the National Action Alliance for Suicide Prevention. (Supplement) | **Total (1 award)** | | **$999,993** |
| **Legislative Authority**: Section 520C of the Public Health Service Act, as amended. | | | |
| **Eligibility**: Limited to the Education Development Center, Inc. Eligibility for this one-year supplemental agreement is being limited because SPRC is currently providing the infrastructure for the Action Alliance and this is the most efficient and effective way to accomplish the goals of advancing the National Strategy for Suicide Prevention. | | | |

Source: GAO analysis of HHS information.

**Table 83: FY 2011 Contract, Suicide Prevention**

| Recipient | Purpose | State | Award (dollars) |
|---|---|---|---|
| Westover Consultants INC | Meeting support | MD | $110,656 |
| **Total (1 award)** | | | **$110,656** |

Source: GAO analysis of HHS information.

# Appendix VI: GAO Contact and Staff Acknowledgments

| | |
|---|---|
| **GAO Contact** | Katherine Iritani, (202) 512-7114 or iritanik@gao.gov |
| **Staff Acknowledgments** | In addition to the contact named above, Kim Yamane, Assistant Director; George Bogart; Carolyn Garvey; Laurie Pachter; and Terry Saiki made key contributions to this report. |

| | |
|---|---|
| **GAO's Mission** | The Government Accountability Office, the audit, evaluation, and investigative arm of Congress, exists to support Congress in meeting its constitutional responsibilities and to help improve the performance and accountability of the federal government for the American people. GAO examines the use of public funds; evaluates federal programs and policies; and provides analyses, recommendations, and other assistance to help Congress make informed oversight, policy, and funding decisions. GAO's commitment to good government is reflected in its core values of accountability, integrity, and reliability. |
| **Obtaining Copies of GAO Reports and Testimony** | The fastest and easiest way to obtain copies of GAO documents at no cost is through GAO's website (www.gao.gov). Each weekday afternoon, GAO posts on its website newly released reports, testimony, and correspondence. To have GAO e-mail you a list of newly posted products, go to www.gao.gov and select "E-mail Updates." |
| **Order by Phone** | The price of each GAO publication reflects GAO's actual cost of production and distribution and depends on the number of pages in the publication and whether the publication is printed in color or black and white. Pricing and ordering information is posted on GAO's website, http://www.gao.gov/ordering.htm.<br><br>Place orders by calling (202) 512-6000, toll free (866) 801-7077, or TDD (202) 512-2537.<br><br>Orders may be paid for using American Express, Discover Card, MasterCard, Visa, check, or money order. Call for additional information. |
| **Connect with GAO** | Connect with GAO on Facebook, Flickr, Twitter, and YouTube.<br>Subscribe to our RSS Feeds or E-mail Updates. Listen to our Podcasts.<br>Visit GAO on the web at www.gao.gov. |
| **To Report Fraud, Waste, and Abuse in Federal Programs** | Contact:<br><br>Website: www.gao.gov/fraudnet/fraudnet.htm<br>E-mail: fraudnet@gao.gov<br>Automated answering system: (800) 424-5454 or (202) 512-7470 |
| **Congressional Relations** | Katherine Siggerud, Managing Director, siggerudk@gao.gov, (202) 512-4400, U.S. Government Accountability Office, 441 G Street NW, Room 7125, Washington, DC 20548 |
| **Public Affairs** | Chuck Young, Managing Director, youngc1@gao.gov, (202) 512-4800 U.S. Government Accountability Office, 441 G Street NW, Room 7149 Washington, DC 20548 |

Please Print on Recycled Paper.

www.ingramcontent.com/pod-product-compliance
Lightning Source LLC
Chambersburg PA
CBHW081130170526
45165CB00008B/2616